MW01119164

Inside—Find the Answers to These Questions and More

- ☑ What supplements may slow the progression of osteoarthritis? (See pages 68 and 90.)

- ☑ How well does glucosamine sulfate reduce arthritis symptoms? (See page 56.)

- ☑ Can chondroitin sulfate protect my joints, and should I combine it with glucosamine? (See page 74.)

- ☑ Is SAMe worth the cost? (See page 93.)

- ☑ What is devil's claw, and can it relieve my pain? (See page 98.)

- ☑ What herbal treatments are available for rheumatoid arthritis? (See page 118.)

- ☑ Does the herb boswellia help rheumatoid arthritis? (See page 119.)

- ☑ How effective is fish oil for rheumatoid arthritis? (See page 107.)

- ☑ Is boron safe to use for osteoarthritis? (See page 135.)

- ☑ What herb is sold as a prescription drug for osteoarthritis? (See page 102.)

THE NATURAL PHARMACIST™ Library

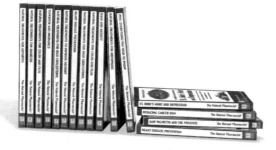

Visit us online at www.TNP.com

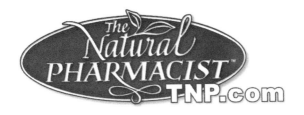

Everything You Need to Know About

Arthritis

Ron Hobbs, N.D.
Gloria Bucco

Series Editors

Steven Bratman, M.D.

David Kroll, Ph.D.

A DIVISION OF PRIMA PUBLISHING

Visit us online at www.TNP.com

Warning—Disclaimer

This book is not intended to provide medical advice and is sold with the understanding that the publisher and the author are not liable for the misconception or misuse of information provided. The author and Prima Publishing shall have neither liability nor responsibility to any person or entity with respect to any loss, damage, or injury caused or alleged to be caused directly or indirectly by the information contained in this book or the use of any products mentioned. Readers should not use any of the products discussed in this book without the advice of a medical professional.

The Food and Drug Administration has not approved the use of any of the natural treatments discussed in this book. This book, and the information contained herein, has not been approved by the Food and Drug Administration.

Pseudonyms are used throughout to protect the privacy of individuals involved.

PRIMA HEALTH and colophon are trademarks of Prima Communications, Inc.

THE NATURAL PHARMACIST™ is a trademark of Prima Communications, Inc.

All products mentioned in this book are trademarks of their respective companies.

Library of Congress Cataloging-in-Publication Data

Hobbs, Ron.
    Arthritis / Ron Hobbs, Gloria Bucco.
      p. cm.—(The natural pharmacist)
    Includes bibliographical references and index.
    ISBN 0-7615-1556-9
    1. Arthritis—Alternative treatment.   2. Arthritis—Popular works.
  3. Naturopathy.   4. Dietary supplements.   I. Hobbs, Ron. II. Title. III. Series.
RC933 .B84   1999
616.7'2206—dc21
                      98-50705
                        CIP
      00 01 02 HH 10 9 8 7 6 5 4
    Printed in the United States of America

Visit us online at www.TNP.com

Contents

What Makes This Book Different?

The interest in natural medicine has never been greater. According to the National Association of Chain Drug Stores, 65 million Americans are using natural supplements, and the number is growing! Yet, it is hard for the consumer to find trustworthy sources for balanced information about this emerging field. Why? Frankly, natural medicine has had a checkered history. From snake oil potions sold at the turn of the century to those books, magazines, and product catalogs that hype miracle cures today, this is a field where exaggerated claims have been the norm. Proponents of natural medicine have tended to abuse science, treating it more as a marketing tool than a means of discovering the truth.

But there is truth to be found. Studies of vitamins, minerals, and other food supplements have been with us since these nutritional substances were first discovered, and the level and quality of this science has grown dramatically in the last 20 years. Herbal medicine has been neglected in the United States, but in Europe, this, the oldest of all healing arts, has been the subject of tremendous and ongoing scientific interest.

At present, for a number of herbs and supplements, it is possible to give reasonably scientific answers to the questions: How well does this work? How safe is it? What types of conditions is it best used for?

THE NATURAL PHARMACIST series is designed to cut through the hype and tell you what we know and what we don't know about popular natural treatments. These books are more conservative than any others available, more honest about the weaknesses of natural approaches, more fair in their comparisons of natural and conventional treatments. You won't find any miracle cures here, but you will discover useful options that can help you become healthier.

Why Choose Natural Treatments?

Although the science behind natural medicine continues to grow, this is still a much less scientifically validated field than conventional medicine. You might ask, "Why should I resort to an herb that is only partly proven, when I could take a drug with solid science behind it?" There are at least three good reasons to consider natural alternatives.

First, some herbs and supplements offer benefits that are not matched by any conventional drug. Vitamin E is a good example. It appears to help prevent prostate cancer, a benefit that no standard medication can claim.

Another example is the herb milk thistle. Studies strongly suggest that this herb can protect the liver from injury. There is no pill or tablet your doctor can prescribe to do the same.

Even if the science behind some of these treatments is less than perfect, when the risks are low and the possible benefit high, a natural treatment may be worth trying. It is a little-known fact that for many conventional treatments the science is less than perfect as well, and physicians must balance uncertain benefits against incompletely understood risks.

A second reason to consider natural therapies is that some may offer benefits comparable to those of drugs with fewer side effects. The herb St. John's wort is a good example. Reasonably strong scientific evidence suggests that this herb is an effective treatment for mild to moderate depression, while producing fewer side effects on average than conventional medications. Saw palmetto for benign enlargement of the prostate, ginkgo for relieving symptoms and perhaps slowing the progression of Alzheimer's disease, and glucosamine for osteoarthritis are other examples. This is not to say that herbs and supplements are completely harmless—they're not—but for most the level of risk is quite low.

Finally, there is a philosophical point to consider. For many people, it "feels" better to use a treatment that comes from nature instead of from a laboratory. Just as you might rather wear all-cotton clothing than polyester, or look at a mountain landscape rather than the skyscrapers of a downtown city, natural treatments may simply feel more compatible with your view of life. We can quibble endlessly about just what "natural" means and whether a certain treatment is "actually" natural or not, but such arguments are beside the point. The difference is in the feeling, and feelings matter. In fact, having a good feeling about taking an herb may lead you to use it more consistently than you would a prescription drug.

Of course, at times synthetic drugs may be necessary and even lifesaving. But on many other occasions it may be quite reasonable to turn to an herb or supplement instead of a drug.

To make good decisions you need good information. Unfortunately, while hundreds of books on alternative medicine are published every year, many are highly misleading. The phrase "studies prove" is often used when the studies in question are so small or so badly conducted that they prove nothing at all. You may even find that the "data" from other books comes from studies with petri dishes and not real people!

You can't even assume that books written by well-known authors are scientifically sound. Many of these authors rely on secondary writers, leading to a game of "telephone," where misconceptions are passed around from book to book. And there's a strong tendency to exaggerate the power of natural remedies, whitewashing them with selective reporting.

THE NATURAL PHARMACIST series gives you the balanced information you need to make informed decisions about your health needs. Setting a new, high standard of accuracy and objectivity, these books take a realistic look at the herbs and supplements you read about in the news. You will encounter both favorable and unfavorable studies in these pages and will learn about both the benefits and the risks of natural treatments.

THE NATURAL PHARMACIST series is the source you can trust.

Steven Bratman, M.D.
David Kroll, Ph.D.

Introduction

All the activities of our daily lives—cooking, dancing, painting a picture, or even just taking a walk or dressing—require the movement of bones in relation to each other. These activities should be easy; however, for those afflicted with arthritis, daily tasks and pleasures can be associated with pain and stiffness. For some, movement is all but impossible.

Arthritis, literally "inflammation of the joints," is a disease of the synovial joints. While arthritis is not a deadly disease, it is, in one form or another, one of the leading causes of disability throughout the world.

The economic costs of arthritis are staggering in terms of medical care and people's inability to work. In 1992, it was estimated that all forms of arthritis cost the American economy about $65 billion. This figure is expected to rise dramatically as the baby boom generation enters its later years. But though the economic cost of arthritis is sky-high, the personal costs may be even greater. How do you put a dollar figure on the ability to dig your own garden or enjoy an afternoon walk?

Entirely satisfactory treatments for arthritis are not yet available. The most common treatment for osteoarthritis, nonsteroidal anti-inflammatory drugs (NSAIDs), predictably damages the stomach lining when used for a long

period of time. Worse yet, NSAIDs may actually accelerate the process of joint damage; further research is
needed on this question, but the possibility is troubling.
New treatments are being investigated and approved; in
fact, as this book goes to press, the U.S. Food and Drug
Administration has approved two new arthritis drugs. But
at present, people with arthritis are faced with difficult
choices among less-than-ideal treatments.

It makes sense that people with arthritis are increasingly open to natural alternative treatments. Any treatment that offers some realistic benefit expands the range
of options. While natural treatments such as glucosamine
sulfate and chondroitin sulfate may not be the "miracle
cures" some advocates claim they are, the research available suggests that they can offer significant help. Not only
can they reduce symptoms, they may also slow or even
stop the usual progressive worsening of osteoarthritis
symptoms, according to preliminary evidence. Many other
treatments can be helpful as well, from S-adenosylmethionine to fish oil.

These natural options are not simply folk medicine or
wishful thinking. All the major treatments discussed in
this book have been subjected to a significant level of formal scientific scrutiny, and many have become standard
treatments in Europe.

In this book we'll explain the evidence for these natural
options and describe their potential benefits and risks.
We'll also tell you what you need to know about dosages
and safety issues.

If you or a loved one have arthritis and want to explore
alternative therapies, this book will give you nonbiased,
scientifically accurate information on the leading natural
treatments. We'll give you the objective information you
need to choose the treatments that will work best for you.

What Is Arthritis?

Evelyn has belonged to a dance club for more than 20 years. She has many close friends in the group, and they are always delighted to see her. Only a few years ago, Evelyn became wheelchair-bound and suffered from such extreme fatigue that she feared she might never dance again. With the help of medical treatment, she has been able to recover much of her health. Yet her friends know they must still hold her hands gently to avoid causing her pain. Evelyn is suffering from arthritis.

Mark has been an athletic guy all his life. In high school and college, he played football. As an adult, he has enjoyed cross-country skiing, hiking, fishing, and rafting. But now, in his 50s, Mark gets out of bed and hobbles to the bathroom every morning. It's only a matter of minutes before his hips loosen up and he's able to walk normally again, but he worries about it getting worse. Mark, too, is suffering from arthritis.

Bonnie is an avid knitter. She began as a teenager, and the hobby has been a great source of pleasure in her life.

1

She knits her own clothing, makes gifts, reads knitting magazines, and attends knitting retreats. But she has to "be good" these days and not knit more than 30 minutes a day, or her fingers become too swollen and painful to move. It's extremely frustrating. Bonnie is also suffering from arthritis.

Some Basic Facts

Arthritis and *rheumatism* are commonly used terms that refer to chronic conditions involving joint pain, stiffness, and swelling that result in limited movement. The term *arthritis* is derived from two Greek words: *arthron,* which means joints, and *itis,* which means inflammation.

As many as one in seven Americans suffers from some form of arthritis.

As many as one in seven Americans suffers from some form of arthritis. In fact, arthritis is the number-one cause of disability in America. In its most advanced stages, arthritis limits everyday activities such as walking, dressing, climbing stairs, and getting in and out of bed. Arthritis can strike at any age (though it's far more common in people over 50), and it restricts activity more often than cardiovascular disease, cancer, or diabetes. For some reason, women are affected more often than men.

There are four common forms of arthritis:

- osteoarthritis
- rheumatoid arthritis
- gout
- juvenile rheumatoid arthritis

Other disorders of the joints and connective tissue include

- lupus
- Sjogren's syndrome
- Reiter's syndrome
- ankylosing spondylitis

For two of these types of arthritis, osteoarthritis and rheumatoid arthritis, there are alternative treatments available that have been scientifically researched and found to have some benefit. Osteoarthritis, the most common form of arthritis, has been treated with glucosamine, chondroitin, S-adenosylmethionine (SAMe), and several types of herbal remedies. As we will see in chapters 5 through 8, there is reasonably good evidence that some of these may offer considerable help for sufferers of this type of arthritis.

Arthritis is the one of the leading causes of disability worldwide.

If you are living with the pain caused by rheumatoid arthritis, chapters 9 and 10 will provide you with information on remedies that may bring additional relief when used with your usual medical treatment.

Osteoarthritis

Physicians and researchers once believed osteoarthritis was an inevitable part of the "wear and tear" of aging. Today we know that even though osteoarthritis is more common in older people (by age 75, almost everyone has some degree of osteoarthritis), it is not simply caused by wear and tear on joints. (See the next chapter for what we now know about the causes of this common disease.)

Janet's Story

Janet is a professional woman in her mid-40s. In the last few years, she began to notice that her knees hurt when she walked downhill or danced. Finally, the discomfort got so bad that she had to give up both her mountain hikes and her dancing—it just hurt too much. Her doctor diagnosed her problem as osteoarthritis and recommended nonsteroidal anti-inflammatory drugs, but they upset Janet's stomach.

Janet mentioned this during a conversation with her mother. Her mother, coincidentally, had just read a book about arthritis and suggested Janet try a combination of chondroitin and glucosamine. "Your father and I have been taking it, and we're both feeling better." Janet decided to try it, too.

After two months of taking the combination of chondroitin and glucosamine, as well as abstaining from dancing, Janet's knees improved enough that she could again begin dancing without needing any aspirin or ibuprofen. In fact, she felt so much better that she began to wonder if it might not be good

Osteoarthritis affects weight-bearing joints, which are the parts of the body that bear the majority of weight, including the hips, knees, and feet. Osteoarthritis also commonly appears in the fingers and spine and is often worse on one side of the body. If you've been noticing pain in your knees as you climb the stairs, or find yourself walking like John Wayne after you've been sitting still for a period of time, you may be getting acquainted with osteoarthritis.

Conventional treatments for osteoarthritis include nonsteroidal anti-inflammatories, or *NSAIDs* (drugs like

for her elderly cat, who at 17 years of age had been having some trouble walking up stairs. She asked her veterinarian, who told her that vets often prescribe this same combination for animals, and he assured her it would be fine to give some to her cat.

Janet's vet thought that the pills she purchased for herself at the pharmacy were likely less expensive than those sold by the veterinary medicine suppliers, so Janet began putting about a fourth of the contents of one capsule into her cat's food in the morning and evening. After a few weeks, she also began seeing a little more bounce in the old cat's steps. She reports that her cat no longer needs her step stool to jump onto the bed at night.

However, as we shall see later in the book, there is no evidence that you need to use a combination of glucosamine and chondroitin. Using only one may be just as effective, and it is certainly safer.

aspirin, ibuprofen, and Naprosyn), as well as acetaminophen, a medication that relieves pain but does not affect inflammation. While these usually reduce symptoms to some extent, none of these conventional treatments slow the progression of osteoarthritis, and some may even speed up its rate of progression.[1,2] In contrast, several natural supplements not only relieve symptoms, but, according to preliminary evidence, may also prevent the disease from getting worse. Chondroitin sulfate has the best evidence for such a "disease-modifying" effect, but glucosamine and S-adenosylmethionine (SAMe) have also

The High Cost of Arthritis

Americans today are living longer. Life expectancy in the United States has nearly doubled since the early 1900s—from 47 years to 76 years. By the year 2025, Americans should be routinely living to the ripe age of 80, according to the World Health Organization. The bulge on census charts known as the postwar baby boom generation is rapidly reaching middle age. In fact, baby boomers have been turning 50 at the rate of one every 7.5 seconds since January 1, 1996. The Census Bureau projects that one in nine baby boomers (9 million of the 78 million people born between 1946 and 1964) will survive into their late 90s, and one in 26 (about 3 million) will reach 100.

been suggested as possibilities. See chapters 5, 6, and 7 for more information on these useful supplements.

Rheumatoid Arthritis

Rheumatoid arthritis may begin with mild joint pain and stiffness; but, unlike osteoarthritis, rheumatoid arthritis may be accompanied by fever, malaise, and loss of appetite and weight. That's because rheumatoid arthritis is an *autoimmune disease.* This means the body begins attacking itself. In the case of rheumatoid arthritis, the body's immune system begins attacking the joints. Rheumatoid arthritis usually affects joints throughout the body and, whereas osteoarthritis often affects one side of the body more than the other, rheumatoid arthritis usually affects the body symmetrically.

Conventional treatment for rheumatoid arthritis consists of two types of treatments: those such as NSAIDs

Now that we are living longer, can we also expect to remain healthy and active longer? The likelihood is very good. But first we will have to jump a few hurdles. One of the highest is a group of diseases commonly referred to as arthritis. By the year 2020, the Centers for Disease Control and Prevention project that arthritis prevalence will increase to 59.4 million Americans, up from 40 million in 1995. This represents 18.2% of the population.

Each year, people make more than 315 million physician visits because of arthritis and are hospitalized for it more than 8 million times. Arthritis costs the nation $65 billion annually in medical costs and lost productivity.

that reduce symptoms, and others that may slow the progression of the disease.

Some natural remedies may also provide relief from the symptoms of rheumatoid arthritis. However, unlike some of the natural treatments for osteoarthritis, none at this time is believed to slow the progression of rheumatoid arthritis. Natural treatments may, however, add additional benefits when used along with conventional medications. For more information, see chapters 9 and 10.

Other Types of Arthritis

Osteoarthritis and rheumatoid arthritis are the most common types of arthritis, but there are other types as well. Unfortunately, at this time there are no scientifically documented alternative therapies for any of the other types of arthritis.

How to Use This Book

If you are suffering from any form of arthritis, this book may be able to provide you with information about your condition. It will be of most use to those with osteoarthritis or rheumatoid arthritis, for which there are some promising alternative treatments.

Keep in mind that no book can substitute for the professional services of a qualified health-care provider.

This book takes a comprehensive look at osteoarthritis and rheumatoid arthritis. We discuss their causes, and—most important—how they can be managed and possibly healed. We will investigate both conventional and alternative medical approaches, where applicable.

Throughout these chapters, we'll provide an objective view of the evidence to enable you to make the most informed decisions possible. None of these treatments is a miracle cure, but some may be very helpful in your search for better health.

Please keep in mind that no book can substitute for the professional services of a qualified health-care provider. Consider the options suggested in this book and discuss them with your physician.

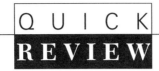

- Arthritis and rheumatism are chronic conditions that involve joint pain, stiffness, and swelling that result in limited movement.
- The four common forms of arthritis are osteoarthritis, rheumatoid arthritis, gout, and juvenile rheumatoid arthritis.
- Osteoarthritis is the most common form of arthritis and affects weight-bearing joints, including the hips, knees, feet, fingers, and spine.
- Rheumatoid arthritis is an autoimmune disease in which the body's immune system attacks the joints. The mild joint pain and stiffness may be accompanied by fever, malaise, and the loss of appetite and weight.
- Alternative treatments for both osteoarthritis and rheumatoid arthritis have been scientifically studied and found to have some benefit.

Osteoarthritis

Rebecca had been a watercolorist for 30 years, so when her fingers began to ache at the end of the day, she was thoroughly alarmed. Her mother's hands had been seriously crippled by osteoarthritis. Rebecca could not stand the thought of losing her ability to paint.

She visited with her family physician, hoping to hear that modern medicine had discovered some new means of dealing with the problem. However, she was disappointed to learn that in two decades, little had changed in this regard. The usual prescription for people with osteoarthritis was still nonsteroidal anti-inflammatory drugs (NSAIDs) such as aspirin, ibuprofen, or some stronger forms not available without a prescription. But because she had a history of ulcers, Rebecca was unable to take NSAID drugs, which are known to contribute to the development of ulcers.

Rebecca was feeling hopeless and a little desperate until she happened to talk to a coworker who suggested looking into some of the alternative therapies. Happily, Rebecca discovered that there is evidence that some of the so-called dietary supplements might give her effective relief from the aching in her joints and could even have what is called a "chondroprotective effect," slowing or preventing her arthritis from worsening.

What Is Osteoarthritis?

Osteoarthritis is an insidious villain that develops gradually, often exhibiting no symptoms for decades. It creeps up on us during our 30s and 40s, usually becoming noticeable in our 50s and 60s.

Also known as *degenerative arthritis* or *degenerative joint disease,* osteoarthritis occurs when cartilage begins to break down and no longer acts as a cushioning pad in the hands, hips, knees, back, and other joints. Without this protective padding, bone will rub against bone. Pain, tenderness, swelling, stiffness, and sometimes deformity can result.

Of the hundreds of types of arthritis that exist, osteoarthritis is by far the most common.

If you suffer from osteoarthritis, you are not alone. The Arthritis Foundation estimates that there are about 15.8 million Americans with osteoarthritis, the majority of them women. In fact, knee arthritis is the most common cause of disability in the developed world.

The condition doesn't affect how long you will live, but it can make everyday activities, and life in general, very uncomfortable for those unlucky enough to have the more serious forms of the disease. But there is some good news: Although osteoarthritis has widely been regarded as an inevitable part of aging, like wrinkles or gray hair, some evidence suggests that it may be preventable.

Protecting Your Joints:
The Search for Chondroprotective Agents

Although standard drugs for osteoarthritis reduce pain, there is worrisome evidence that they may contribute to the problem by interfering with the efforts of cartilage to repair itself.[1,2] When this was discovered, researchers in Europe began to look for substances that could protect cartilage from further harm. The term for such a substance is a "chondroprotective agent." The concept of chondroprotective agents has not been widely accepted among U.S. physicians, although veterinarians in the United States have begun to use it.

A number of substances have been proposed as chondroprotective agents. The reasoning behind two of them, glucosamine and chondroitin, is almost embarrassingly simple: They

Who Is Affected by Osteoarthritis?

By age 65, about 70% of all people have x-ray evidence of osteoarthritis in their weight-bearing joints. About 100,000 people in the United States suffer from hip or knee arthritis that makes it impossible to walk unassisted from their bed to the bathroom. The disease tends to develop at an earlier age in males. Under the age of 45, symptomatic osteoarthritis is more common in men; between the ages of 45 and 55, and men and women are equally affected. After 55, osteoarthritis is more common in women.[3]

contain raw materials necessary for rebuilding cartilage. Hypothetically, supplying extra amounts of these raw materials may enable cartilage to repair itself faster.

Another proposed chondroprotective agent, S-adenosylmethionine, is believed to help cartilage repair and possibly exert other helpful effects.

If chondroprotective agents live up to their name, they might even stop osteoarthritis from following its natural course and becoming worse with time. If so, they could be called "disease-modifying drugs," unlike other treatments that just reduce symptoms temporarily. More research, however, is necessary before we can say for sure that chondroprotective agents really work this way.

Signs and Symptoms of Osteoarthritis

You may have osteoarthritis and not even know it. Osteoarthritis doesn't make you feel "sick." You won't have a fever, and you won't lose weight. In fact, you may be unaware of the condition until it shows up in an x ray. When symptoms do begin to occur, they are usually mild at first and can include morning stiffness that disappears quickly.

Another warning sign of osteoarthritis is pain. You may be surprised by a pain in one or both knees when you rise from a sitting position. Or you may experience pain in a joint after you overuse it or use it after being inactive for a while.

Osteoarthritis: An Ancient Problem

Osteoarthritis is not a twentieth-century disease. Far from it. Fossilized bones show that Ice Age cave people suffered from osteoarthritis. Signs of osteoarthritis have also been found in Egyptian and Peruvian mummies and in ancient Native American and Roman remains.

Two members of a herd of the dinosaur known as Iguanadon, which are mounted in a Brussels museum, show clear signs of osteoarthritis of the ankle.[4]

Symptoms differ depending on which joint is affected. Osteoarthritis of the hands leads to pain and limited use. Osteoarthritis in the knees produces pain, swelling, and instability. Osteoarthritis of the hip causes local pain and a limp. Slow deterioration of discs between the bones along the spine can lead to back and neck stiffness.

As the disease advances, you may experience pain when moving the affected joint. The pain might be worse during periods of activity and may abate when you are at rest. For some, osteoarthritis never gets beyond this point. For others, symptoms gradually worsen until they eventually limit daily activities such as walking, climbing stairs, or typing.

You may also begin to lose *range of motion*—how far one part of your body can move while the rest of you is holding still. With osteoarthritis, that distance may decrease. You may not be able to turn your head as far to the side as you once could or lift your leg as high. This can translate into inconvenience in daily living: You may find it more difficult to check behind you for oncoming traffic while driving, or climb a stepladder to change a light bulb.

Which Joints Are Usually Affected?

Weight-bearing joints are the most susceptible to osteoarthritis, and the disease most often occurs in the knees, hips, and feet. It can also manifest in the fingers and spine. It's uncommon, however, for osteoarthritis to affect the jaw, shoulders, elbows, wrists, or ankles, unless you've been injured or placed unusual stress on one of these joints.

Knees, which bear the weight of the entire body, are among the body's most unstable joints. This is because knee joints must be supported by ligaments and cartilage. If either of these is damaged, the knee has a limited potential to repair itself because ligaments and cartilage are slow to heal.

In some cases of osteoarthritis, finger joints may feel tender, painful, or stiff. Bony knobs called "nodes" may form and enlarge finger joints. *Heberden's nodes,* the most common type, affect the joints at the end of the fingers. This type of node takes years to appear and tends to run in families, affecting more women than men.

Weight-bearing joints are the most susceptible to osteoarthritis, and the disease most often occurs in the knees, hips, and feet.

What Causes Osteoarthritis?

Although once thought of as a wear-and-tear disease, a new theory holds that osteoarthritis is a chemical disease of cartilage, the material that covers the ends of the bones where they join. Cartilage has a high water content and is mostly made up of a gel-like protein called

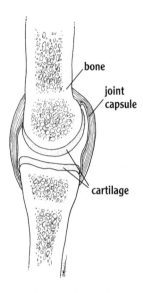

Figure 1. *Cartilage cushions the bones*

collagen. Cartilage acts as a shock absorber, cushioning the bones and preventing them from grinding against each other as they move (see figure 1). As we'll soon see, osteoarthritis may be the result of an imbalance in the normal breakdown and buildup of cartilage.

One item of evidence has helped overturn the wear-and-tear theory: Joints have a low friction level, so they don't wear out by themselves unless they are used excessively or are injured.[5] Also, while osteoarthritis does occur more frequently in joints that have been stressed or damaged, it can also occur in uninjured joints. Furthermore, osteoarthritis frequently develops in many joints at the same time, often on both sides of the body symmetrically, even when there is no reason to believe that joints on both sides of the body have been subjected to equal amounts of wear and tear.

Another intriguing clue is that osteoarthritis of the knee is commonly (and mysteriously) associated with osteoarthritis of the hands. These factors as well as others have led to the suggestion that osteoarthritis may actually be a systemic, or body-wide, disease of the cartilage.

Cartilage is primarily made of two types of substances: *proteoglycans* and *collagen.* Proteoglycans stiffen the tissue and give it the ability to withstand the pressure placed on joints, for instance when you are lifting heavy objects. Collagen fibers give it strength to hold together even when stretched and ground between the bones it protects.

Osteoarthritis may be the result of an imbalance in the normal breakdown and buildup of cartilage.

The cartilage in your body is constantly being turned over by a balance of forces that both break it down and rebuild it. One prevailing theory suggests that osteoarthritis may represent a situation in which the forces that break down cartilage get out of hand for reasons that are unknown. We do know that substances called *metalloproteinases, plasmin,* and *cathepsins* all play a role in destroying cartilage, and they are found in increased amounts in the joints of those suffering from osteoarthritis. There is some evidence that *chondroitin,* a supplement we'll discuss in more detail in chapter 6, may slow joint deterioration by interfering with enzymes that help the breaking-down process.

The first changes seen in osteoarthritis involve an abnormality of cartilage. These abnormalities include subtle disruptions in the network of fibers that make up the cartilage. In response to the damage, rebuilding mechanisms take effect, increasing production of collagen and proteoglycans.

Certain natural supplements, such as glucosamine, S-adenosylmethionine, and chondroitin, may be able to support this rebuilding mechanism.

Even after osteoarthritis has begun, these compensating mechanisms can keep the joint functioning well for several years. Because the cartilage has been damaged, it may thicken, but it still functions. The phase of osteoarthritis during which the joint remains functioning is called "compensated" or "stabilized" osteoarthritis. Eventually, however, unaided building forces cannot keep up with destructive ones, and what is called "end-stage" osteoarthritis develops. End-stage osteoarthritis results in the all-too-familiar picture of arthritic pain and impaired joint function.

In chapters 5 through 8 and 11, we'll discuss the ways certain natural treatments may be able to reduce the symptoms of osteoarthritis. We'll also explore exciting new evidence that some natural treatments may even slow the deterioration of the joints, actually changing the progress of the disease. This, as we'll discuss in chapter 4, is something that none of the conventional medicines available for osteoarthritis are able to do.

Factors That Influence Osteoarthritis

In the search for clues to solve the mystery of why osteoarthritis occurs, researchers look at the factors that influence the development of the disease. We have already noted that the statistical risk of developing osteoarthritis increases with age and is higher for women than for men. This was once attributed to a lifetime of wear and tear, but as we've seen, present thinking suggests that there may be other causes. However, we don't know precisely what they are.

The following factors have been shown to have an impact on the incidence or severity of osteoarthritis:

- Injuries
- Heredity
- Obesity
- Occupation

Injuries

When a joint has been damaged by injury, severe overuse, or another disease, arthritis symptoms may develop over time. This is called *secondary arthritis*. (*Primary arthritis* is the ordinary kind that arises seemingly from nowhere.)

Exercise in general promotes health, and some exercise may actually strengthen joints and muscles. This is great, because some evidence shows that weak muscles can lead to osteoarthritis.[6] Weakness in the thigh muscles, for instance, puts greater stress on the knee joint, setting up the process of wear and tear. Strengthening these muscles might help prevent osteoarthritis, or at least keep it from progressing as quickly. However, excessive use of parts of the body can cause osteoarthritis symptoms to begin earlier in life.

It's important to note that recreational sports at a reasonable level are not likely to be harmful for most people.[7] Joints that are healthy to begin with appear to tolerate prolonged, vigorous, low-impact exercise without accelerated development of osteoarthritis. However, if you have already suffered damage to a joint, ligament, or tendon, you may need to be especially careful.[8,9] Your doctor should be able to suggest appropriate sports and a good level of activity.

Heredity

Genetics appears to play a role in the development of osteoarthritis in the hands. However, it's a modest role. Just because your mother had hand arthritis doesn't mean you and your siblings will too. Most likely, a combination of genetic susceptibility *and* other unidentified factors in the environment must all be present at the same time if you're to develop the disease.

Obesity

After the age of 65, the majority of adults in the industrialized world are obese, and obesity appears to be a risk factor for knee osteoarthritis.[10] Unlike aging and genetics, this is one risk factor we can control. Losing weight will not only prolong your life, it will reduce the risk of living with serious discomfort.

Occupation

Certain job-related activities continued for many years can induce osteoarthritis in specific joints, most likely because of repeated injuries.[11] Some well-studied examples include osteoarthritis of the knees and spine in miners, osteoarthritis of the hip in farmers, and increased rates of osteoarthritis in the upper joints of pneumatic-drill operators. If you're in a profession that severely stresses your joints, you might be particularly interested to know that chondroitin and other "chondroprotective" substances may help prevent arthritis from developing or progressing.

Weather

Many people suffering from osteoarthritis swear that weather conditions influence their joint pain. So far, science can offer no proof that this is true, nor can it explain why this seems to happen. Few studies have been published on the subject, and they offer differing opinions.[12] Physicians agree, however, that for those who believe weather can influence their pain, even though the causes remain unknown, the effect is real. Unfortunately, there isn't much you can do about this risk factor except retire to a warm climate.

Diagnosing Osteoarthritis

As previously mentioned, you may have osteoarthritis and not even know it. A diagnosis of osteoarthritis is usually made based on a physical exam and the patient's history of osteoarthritis-related symptoms. Physicians often order x rays to confirm their diagnosis, looking for such signs as bony spurs and evidence of cartilage destruction.

A diagnosis of osteoarthritis is usually based on a physical exam and the patient's history of symptoms. Doctors often order x rays to confirm their diagnosis.

In later chapters, we'll discuss the conventional treatments used for the various types of arthritis, as well as some promising alternative therapies. If you suffer from symptoms of osteoarthritis, you may be especially interested in the information provided in chapters 5 through 8 as well as the evidence shown for the benefits of fruits and vegetables discussed in chapter 12.

In the next chapter, we'll look at the causes and symptoms of rheumatoid arthritis, the second-most common type of arthritis.

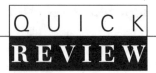

- Osteoarthritis is the most common form of arthritis. It occurs when the cartilage between bones breaks down.
- The symptoms of osteoarthritis include pain, stiffness, limited range of motion, and sometimes inflammation.
- No one is certain what causes osteoarthritis. However, researchers believe injury, heredity, obesity, and certain occupations can increase the risk of developing osteoarthritis.
- Low-impact exercises and sports do not appear to increase the risk of developing osteoarthritis in normal, healthy joints.
- Obesity is one health factor we can change to lesson our risk of osteoarthritis.

CHAPTER
THREE

Rheumatoid Arthritis

At first, Carol believed she had some kind of flu. She was tired, felt feverish, and her joints ached. She thought it would probably go away in a few days, though, and since she didn't have any other symptoms, she didn't think she should call in sick to work. But after a week had passed, she still wasn't feeling better.

One day after lunch, her supervisor came to her office cubicle and found her sleeping with her head cradled in her arms on the desk. Embarrassed, she explained how she'd been feeling, and her supervisor suggested she see her doctor.

Carol's doctor examined her but didn't find anything obvious. He ordered the standard lab tests, but they revealed only one unusual finding: Carol had anemia. He prescribed iron supplements, hoping they would at least get rid of her fatigue.

Several weeks later, however, her anemia was unimproved. Then Carol developed more severe pain in the joints of her hands and wrists. They began to swell and became so sore she could barely move them.

At this point, her physician recognized that Carol might be suffering from rheumatoid arthritis. He ordered another blood test to see if her blood contained rheumatoid factor (an antibody present in the blood when rheumatoid arthritis is present). This test came back positive. At the final visit he found flat nodules under the skin near her elbows. Putting all the pieces together, her doctor decided she did indeed have rheumatoid arthritis. At last, Carol had a diagnosis. She finally knew what she was fighting. As always, that's the first step toward winning.

What Is Rheumatoid Arthritis?

Rheumatoid arthritis is similar to osteoarthritis in many ways, but it differs in at least two important respects.

Rheumatoid arthritis is an autoimmune disease: The body turns on itself and attacks its own tissues, producing severe and painful inflammation.

First, rheumatoid arthritis is an autoimmune disease. This means that the body turns on itself and attacks its own tissues, producing the severe and painful inflammation that is the hallmark of this disease.

Second, although both osteoarthritis and rheumatoid arthritis affect the joints, osteoarthritis begins by attacking the cartilage. Rheumatoid arthritis begins by attacking a part of the joint called the *synovial membrane.*

The synovial membrane is a smooth, thin layer of tissue that surrounds each joint in the body. It secretes a lubricant called *syn-*

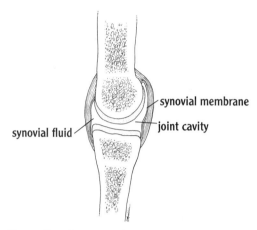

Figure 2. *The synovial membrane and fluid allow the joint to move smoothly*

ovial fluid into the joint cavity. The synovial membrane and synovial fluid allow the joints to move with very little friction (see figure 2). The fluid also carries nutrients to the bones and cartilage inside the capsule.

Who Is Affected by Rheumatoid Arthritis?

Rheumatoid arthritis affects 1 to 2% of the population. Prior to menopause, women develop it about two to three times more often than men, but postmenopausally, the rates even out. It usually appears between 20 and 50 years of age, but it can begin at any age. Rheumatoid arthritis is observed throughout the world and affects all races. For some reason, its incidence and severity seem to be less in rural sub-Saharan Africa[1] and in the Inuit (Eskimos).[2] (See chapter 9 for a discussion of how the Inuit might be protected against rheumatoid arthritis.)

Signs and Symptoms

Rheumatoid arthritis may begin subtly, affecting only a few joints, or it may begin with a sudden flare-up involving many joints. Often, the first sign of rheumatoid arthritis is

nonspecific symptoms such as fatigue, a low-grade fever, and loss of appetite and weight. Weakness and a general malaise may continue throughout the course of the illness, often being most pronounced in the early afternoon.

Rheumatoid arthritis affects 1 to 2% of the population.

Rheumatoid arthritis varies in intensity from person to person. It can range from mild, chronic discomfort to severe pain with limited motion and deformity. Rheumatoid arthritis usually attacks the hands and feet, causing inflammation that results in swelling, pain, and often, eventual destruction of the tissue that lines and cushions joints. The cause of this inflammation is unknown, but we do know it attacks in a symmetrical pattern—that is, it affects the same joint on both sides of the body.

Pain and Stiffness

The classic symptom of rheumatoid arthritis is morning joint pain and stiffness that eases as the day progresses—the so-called rusty gate syndrome. Pain and stiffness also occur after intense activity. These periods of pain and stiffness will generally lengthen as the disease becomes more active.

Typically, small joints in the fingers, toes, hands, feet, wrists, elbows, and ankles become inflamed first. They may become red, warm, and swollen, and the skin over the joint may take on a ruddy, purplish hue. Infected joints usually enlarge and can quickly become deformed. They may also "freeze" in one position, temporarily or permanently.

Rheumatoid Nodules

Another characteristic of rheumatoid arthritis is formation of *rheumatoid nodules,* small lumps of tissue that form under the skin, usually near the joints. These nodules are found in 30 to 40% of patients.

Other Symptoms

Other symptoms may include carpal tunnel syndrome (a common, painful compression of a nerve going into the hand, most recognized as a work-related injury caused by repetitive motion); Sjogren's syndrome (extreme dryness of the eyes, mouth, and other mucous membranes); cysts (which can rupture) located behind affected knees (where they can cause pain and swelling in the lower legs); and atrophy of the skin and muscles around affected joints.

Often, the first sign of rheumatoid arthritis is non-specific symptoms such as fatigue, a low-grade fever, and loss of appetite and weight.

As was the case with Carol, whose story began this chapter, about one-quarter of rheumatoid arthritis patients also develop anemia—a shortage of red blood cells, which can cause feelings of fatigue. Rheumatoid arthritis may also produce a low-grade fever and occasionally an inflammation of blood vessels (*vasculitis*) that causes nerve damage or leg sores (*ulcers*). Some people will develop swollen lymph nodes.

Infrequent Complications of Rheumatoid Arthritis

Infrequently, rheumatoid arthritis may cause more serious problems. These include inflammation of the heart or the membrane covering the heart (a condition known as *pericarditis*), an enlarged spleen, inflammation of the membranes surrounding the lung (a condition called *pleurisy*), and inflammation of the outer layers of the eye, which can lead to blindness.

The Natural Course of Rheumatoid Arthritis

About 10% of patients diagnosed with rheumatoid arthritis recover fully within 1 year. Another 40 to 65% go into remission within 2 years.[3] People in these two groups usually have mild symptoms.

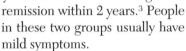

If rheumatoid arthritis remains active for more than 2 years, there is a much greater chance of significant joint deformity. The disease will progress in approximately one half of the people who suffer from rheumatoid arthritis, requiring aggressive therapy. At least 1 in 10 people with rheumatoid arthritis eventually become disabled.[4] Doctors are beginning to use genetic markers and other methods to identify early on those patients whose disease may progress, justifying more aggressive treatment.[5]

> **About 10% of patients diagnosed with rheumatoid arthritis experience complete remission within 1 year. Another 40 to 65% go into remission within 2 years.**

Causes of Rheumatoid Arthritis

Rheumatoid arthritis is an autoimmune disease. In this case, the body's immune system attacks the synovial membrane (the smooth tissue that surrounds your body's joints) as though it were a virus or bacteria. It's a bit like so-called friendly fire in a war. Instead of bullets and

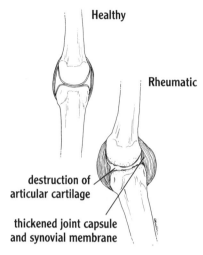

Figure 3. *A healthy joint versus a rheumatic one*

bombs hitting your troops, white blood cells attack the synovial membrane with free radicals and other destructive chemicals. Under the onslaught, the synovial membrane becomes inflamed—red, hot, swollen, and painful.

Your immune system can't eliminate all the parts of your body that it sees as invaders (as it does with viruses or other foreign bodies), so the inflammation continues and may become chronic, resulting in significant damage.

The damaged synovial membrane then begins to grow, thickening so much that it impinges on the cartilage of the joint. This overgrown membrane is referred to as a *pannus.* As the tissue continues to increase in size, it squeezes cartilage and bones within the joint, causing more damage (see figure 3). Enzymes and growth factors released by the synovial membrane and white blood cells also cause joint deterioration, breaking down some tissues and encouraging others to grow too fast, respectively. Finally, the pannus can also directly limit joint motion simply by being in the way.

The autoimmune process of rheumatoid arthritis is not, however, restricted only to the joints. The whole body may be involved, leading to the symptoms of fatigue, malaise, weight loss, weakness, and anemia described earlier.

Factors That Influence Rheumatoid Arthritis

As with osteoarthritis, there are some factors that are known to influence the development of rheumatoid arthritis. The most prominent factors are:

- Heredity
- Microorganisms

Heredity

There seems to be a genetic component to rheumatoid arthritis.[6] For example, severe rheumatoid arthritis is found at about four times the expected rate in first-degree relatives (parents, siblings) of those who suffer from the disease. Additionally, researchers at the Mayo Clinic found that people with rheumatoid arthritis who have inherited certain gene markers from both their parents (rather than just one parent) have a higher risk of developing a severe form of the disease (which could involve internal organs as well as joints).[7] This finding is significant because it can lead to identification and early treatment of people known to be at higher risk for developing more severe cases of rheumatoid arthritis.

However, not everyone with the gene markers for rheumatoid arthritis develops the disease. Thus these genes appear to only predispose a person to rheumatoid arthritis; they don't create it. Environment must also play a role.

Microorganisms

Most treatments for rheumatoid arthritis work by directly reducing inflammation or by toning down the ferocity of the body's attack against itself. A completely different approach involves the use of antibiotics. This method is based on theories that microorganisms such as bacteria, fungi, protozoa, or viruses may play a role in rheumatoid arthritis.[8]

One school of thought maintains that a microorganism infects the synovial tissue, causing damage and inflammation. Another speculates that the microorganism might induce an immune response against a joint by altering it somewhat or revealing normally hidden proteins.[9] The body may regard these altered or previously hidden proteins as invaders. Think of this as flying an enemy flag in the middle of your own troops.

Diagnosing Rheumatoid Arthritis

Rheumatoid arthritis leads to severe disability in more than 50% of cases within 5 years. Further, the time from onset of symptoms to joint destruction is sometimes measured in months rather than years. Clearly, there is some urgency to diagnose it immediately.[10]

However, distinguishing rheumatoid arthritis from other similar diseases can be tricky. Many conditions resemble rheumatoid arthritis. These include osteoarthritis, acute rheumatic fever, Lyme disease, gout, Reiter's syndrome (an arthritic disorder in men that may result from a virus or fungal infection), and ankylosing spondylitis (a long-term inflammatory disease of unknown origin). So, due to rheumatoid arthritis's subtle and confounding first symptoms, initiation of effective therapy often comes later rather than sooner, resulting in irreversible joint destruction.[11]

A physician will begin by taking a medical history and conducting a physical exam to rule out other possible causes of symptoms. Lab tests, x rays, examination of a joint fluid sample, and possibly a biopsy (removal of a tissue sample for examination under a microscope) of rheumatoid

Elaine, Tom, and Abbey: Three Approaches to Treating Rheumatoid Arthritis

Elaine's rheumatoid arthritis showed up for the first time when she was about 25, but it took almost a year for her to get a diagnosis. The symptoms would come and go; sometimes she felt fine, but then her joints would flare up, especially in her knees. The symptoms were never severe, but they were annoying.

On the advice of her physician, Elaine began to take anti-inflammatories and occasionally steroids. She has found considerable relief from her symptoms, and she can frequently stop taking any medication when her symptoms die down. She might also consider trying fish oil, as described in chapter 9.

Tom had a different experience with his rheumatoid arthritis. His level of pain was severe, often so intense that he couldn't walk. His doctor was concerned that he might have a serious form of rheumatoid arthritis and recommended he use the drug methotrexate. As we shall see in chapter 4, methotrexate is be-

nodules may be necessary to pin down a diagnosis. Examination of joint fluid usually reflects the degree of inflammation. X-ray findings usually show soft tissue swelling, erosion of cartilage, and joint-space narrowing.

Identification of an antibody in the blood called *rheumatoid factor* is a central diagnostic tool for rheumatoid arthritis. Usually, the higher the level of rheumatoid factor in the blood, the more severe the rheumatoid arthritis and the poorer the prognosis. However, this is not a perfect test. As many as 3 out of 10 rheumatoid arthritis patients do not have detectable rheumatoid factor. Fur-

lieved to modify the course of rheumatoid arthritis, possibly preventing permanent joint damage.

Abbey tried everything the doctor suggested for her rheumatoid arthritis, but her flare-ups were still making her life miserable. Then she read an article about using antibiotic therapy. Though her doctor was not convinced that treating Abbey with antibiotics made sense, she agreed to give Abbey a prescription for minocycline simply because nothing else had worked.

Although Abbey's doctor still expresses her doubts that Abbey's subsequent pain relief is anything but a placebo effect, Abbey believes the antibiotics are working to keep her disease in remission.

Rheumatoid arthritis affects people in different ways, and each person appears to respond to treatments differently as well. Chapters 9 through 12 will offer some suggestions that may be helpful for you to try if you are living with rheumatoid arthritis.

thermore, this antibody can also occur in several other disorders, such as chronic liver disease. To complicate matters even more, some people have this factor without any evidence of disease, while others have the disease without showing the factor.

The conventional treatments used for rheumatoid arthritis will be discussed in more depth in chapter 4. Chapters 9 through 12 offer some additional alternative approaches that may help to relieve the discomfort of rheumatoid arthritis when used in conjunction with conventional medicines.

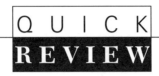

- Rheumatoid arthritis is an autoimmune disease in which the immune system attacks the synovial membrane located in the body's joints.

- It affects more premenopausal women than men, but affects postmenopausal women at approximately the same rate as men.

- Rheumatoid arthritis is characterized by symmetrical inflammation of joints that can result in damage to cartilage, bones, tendons, and ligaments.

- Researchers have not determined exactly what causes the inflammation associated with the disease.

- The autoimmune process of rheumatoid arthritis is not restricted to the joints. The entire body may become involved, leading to symptoms of fatigue, malaise, weight loss, weakness, and anemia.

- Rheumatoid arthritis's symptoms can mimic those of other diseases, including osteoarthritis, acute rheumatic fever, Lyme disease, gout, Reiter's syndrome, and ankylosing spondylitis.

- In addition to evaluating a patient's symptoms and medical history, blood tests and x rays may be necessary to diagnose rheumatoid arthritis.

Conventional Treatments for Arthritis

T he goals of conventional treatments for all types of arthritis focus on relieving pain, reducing inflammation, maintaining normal function, and preventing deformities. Many treatments are used to accomplish these goals, including medications, physical therapy, and surgery. This chapter will address the many available conventional medications.

The most widespread group of medications used to manage arthritis is nonsteroidal anti-inflammatory drugs, or NSAIDs. NSAIDs are the most commonly prescribed class of drugs in the United States—between 70 and 75 million prescriptions are written annually. Aspirin, ibuprofen (Advil, Motrin), naproxen (Aleve, Naprosyn, Naprelan), and ketoprofen (Actron, Orudis KT) are common NSAIDs, but there are many others. (Table 1 lists arthritis medications by category.) NSAIDs are the primary treatment for osteoarthritis and are also used in mild cases of rheumatoid arthritis. They work both by relieving pain and controlling inflammation. However, they do not

Table 1. Medications Used for Arthritis

Brand Name	generic name
Analgesics	
Capzasin P	capsaicin (topical)
Tylenol	acetaminophen
Ultram	tramadol
Zostrix	capsaicin (topical)
NSAIDs	
Actron	ketoprofen
Advil	ibuprofen
Aleve	naproxen sodium
Anaprox	naproxen sodium
Ansaid	flurbiprofen
Arthrotec	diclofenac sodium and misoprostol
Azulfidine	sulfasalazine
Bayer Arthritis	aspirin
Cataflam	diclofenac potassium
Celebrex	celecoxib
Clinoril	sulindac
Daypro	oxaprozin
Disalcid	salsalate
Dolobid	diflunisal
Easprin	aspirin
Ecotrin	aspirin
Feldene	piroxicam
Indocin	indomethacin
Lodine	etodolac
Meclomen	meclofenamate sodium
Motrin	ibuprofen
Nalfon	fenoprofen calcium
Naprelan	naproxen
Naprosyn	naproxen
Nuprin	ibuprofen
Orudis	ketoprofen
Oruvail	ketoprofen

Table 1. Medications Used for Arthritis *(continued)*

Brand Name	generic name
Relafen	nabumetone
Salflex	salsalate
Tolectin	tolmetin
Trilisate	salicylate
Voltaren	diclofenac sodium

Corticosteroids

Aristocort	triamcinolone
Cortef	hydrocortisone
Deltasone	prednisone
Medrol	methylpredisolone
Prelone	prednisolone

DMARDs

ANTIMALARIALS

Plaquenil	hydroxychloroquine sulfate

GOLD SALTS

Myochrysine	gold sodium thiomalate (injectable)
Ridaura	auranofin (oral gold)
Solganol	aurothioglucose (injectable)

CHELATING AGENTS

Cuprimine	penicillamine
Depen	penicillamine

IMMUNE SUPPRESSANTS

Arava	leflunomide
Imuran	azathioprine
Neoral	cyclosporine
Rheumatrex	methotrexate
Sandimmune	cyclosporine

Antibiotics

Minocin	minocycline

Other

Enbrel	etanercept

Dorothy's Story

Dorothy was diagnosed with osteoarthritis 8 months ago. Her left knee had begun to hurt so badly that she found it quite difficult to walk her dogs, let alone play tennis, her favorite sport. Her doctor placed her on a nonsteroidal anti-inflammatory called piroxicam. It dramatically helped her knee pain, but over time she gradually developed stomach upset. She didn't want to tell her doctor because she greatly appreciated the pain relief it offered. However, her stomach pain finally became too severe to ignore. She was waking up every night, getting stomachaches all afternoon, and taking antacids throughout the day.

When she finally told her doctor, he was very alarmed by her story and told her to stop the piroxicam at once. He then gave her a prescription for the stomach medication prilosec and told her that if the pain didn't go away rapidly he wanted to perform a test to see if she had an ulcer.

slow down the progression of rheumatoid arthritis; and as we shall see, there is some evidence that they may actually speed the progression of osteoarthritis.

Another category of drugs used to manage arthritis pain is analgesics, like Tylenol (acetaminophen) and Ultram (tramadol). These can also be used for any type of arthritis. They reduce pain but do not affect inflammation nor alter the course of the disease.

Many other drugs are available, particularly for the treatment of rheumatoid arthritis. We will discuss these in the last portion of this chapter.

All these drugs, including over-the-counter acetaminophen and NSAIDs, can be quite useful, but they also

Fortunately, after 2 weeks, the stomach discomfort was almost entirely gone. Just as she had feared, however, her knee pain came back with a vengeance. Her doctor told her quite frankly that he was in a bit of a quandary. They could try a different type of anti-inflammatory drug; but her reaction to the first one had been so severe, he felt concerned she might develop an ulcer. She could take Tylenol, but he doubted that it would be strong enough. The other possibility was to combine an anti-inflammatory drug with another drug to help protect her stomach lining.

Unfortunately, neither she nor her doctor knew that there were other options. In chapters 5 through 8 and 11, we'll describe some safe, natural treatments that may relieve arthritis and perhaps even slow down its natural progression.

have potential side effects ranging from mild to serious to life threatening. In this chapter, we'll examine conventional approaches to arthritis treatment, how the approaches affect arthritis, and what they do to the body. The remaining chapters will address some of the alternative treatments available for arthritis.

NSAIDs: Nonsteroidal Anti-Inflammatory Drugs

Nonsteroidal anti-inflammatory drugs are aptly named: They are not steroids, yet they control certain forms of inflammation. Aspirin was the first NSAID. In recent decades, numerous synthetic variations on the theme have been developed. Besides relieving inflammation, these medications also directly reduce pain.

NSAIDs are quite effective for osteoarthritis, substantially reducing pain and increasing mobility. They are also moderately helpful in the early stages of rheumatoid arthritis. However, all presently available NSAIDs produce a significant

NSAIDs are anti-inflammatory drugs that also reduce pain.

degree of stomach irritation that frequently complicates their use. (New NSAIDs under development at the time of this writing, called COX-2 inhibitors, may reduce or eliminate this problem. The first COX-2 inhibitor, called Celebrex, was approved by the FDA in early 1999.) NSAIDs generally carry the warning that they should be taken with food to minimize stomach

upset, but this is frequently not effective. Some degree of gastrointestinal bleeding occurs in over half of the people taking NSAIDs,[1] and continued use can lead to ulcers.

Normally, stomach pain develops as a warning sign long before an ulcer develops. However, with NSAIDs, severe stomach damage can occur without significant discomfort, and an ulcer may go all the way through the stomach lining without any preceding symptoms. In 1989 alone, there were 2,600 deaths and 20,000 hospitalizations attributed to NSAID-related stomach injury in patients with rheumatoid arthritis.[2]

Unfortunately, NSAIDs cause stomach ulcers through a process closely related to how they function. NSAIDs block the synthesis of hormone-like substances known as *prostaglandins*. Since prostaglandins play a major role in inflammation, NSAIDs' effect on prostaglandins is presumed to be one of the major ways in which NSAIDs help control inflammation, although there are other possible mechanisms as well.

But prostaglandins also play a role in protecting the lining of the stomach from acids. By destroying prostaglandins, NSAIDs break down the protective mucus barrier of the stomach lining, allowing acid to make its way into the stomach wall itself. NSAIDs can also damage other areas of the digestive tract.[3] Special "designer" NSAIDs currently under development more specifically target prostaglandins outside the stomach. These drugs may therefore be less likely to cause stomach problems, although this has not yet been proven.

Elderly people, people taking corticosteroids (such as prednisone), and people with a history of stomach ulcers, alcoholism, or stomach upset with NSAIDs are at higher risk of developing ulcers. To complicate matters, standard anti-ulcer medications such as Zantac and Pepcid do not prevent NSAID-induced ulcers. One special drug, misoprostol (Cytotec), does offer some protection, but it frequently produces a terrific case of diarrhea.

Besides severe stomach injury, NSAIDs can also cause kidney damage and, occasionally, liver injury. Furthermore, there is also some evidence (but no absolute proof) that NSAIDs impair the body's ability to repair cartilage and may also damage cartilage directly.[4] The net effect may be to accelerate the progression of joint damage.[5] This is particularly worrisome for a drug prescribed for arthritis!

In contrast, some of the alternative treatments to be discussed in subsequent chapters, especially chondroitin sulfate, may actually help cartilage regenerate. And none of them is associated with severe side effects.

Analgesics: Pain-Relieving Drugs

As we mentioned above, NSAIDs are both anti-inflammatory and analgesic (pain-relieving) drugs. Acetaminophen, on the other hand, is purely an analgesic.

Because it produces no effect on prostaglandins, it does not cause stomach irritation. Acetaminophen appears to be about as effective as low doses of NSAIDs.[6] However, it seldom provides adequate relief in any but the mild stages of arthritis.

The maximum daily dosage of acetaminophen is 4,000 mg.[7] If this dosage is exceeded, even by a fairly small amount, liver damage is not only possible but likely. Use of acetaminophen with alcohol has been found to increase the risk of liver injury dramatically.

NSAIDs can cause stomach ulcers.

Opiate drugs like codeine and Percodan are more powerful analgesics than Tylenol. Because they are highly addictive, however, they are seldom used for arthritis. A newer, non-opiate analgesic called tramadol (Ultram) is also being used, but at higher doses it can act like an opiate, and recent trends suggest that it also has the potential to be abused.

Corticosteroids

Corticosteroids such as prednisone are highly effective drugs for suppressing the immune system and reducing general inflammation in the body. This combination makes them highly effective for suppressing the inflammatory symptoms of rheumatoid arthritis.

Unfortunately, while corticosteroids are safe in the short term, long-term treatment inevitably causes severe problems. These include dramatic osteoporosis (thinning of the bones), poor wound healing, easy bruising, high blood pressure, elevated blood sugar levels possibly leading to diabetes, and cataracts. Corticosteroids can decrease bone mass by as much as 10 to 20% in the first 6 months of therapy.[8] They are also associated with weight gain, which can become a serious problem. In some cases, a high dosage of steroids can be given intermittently and then tapered off, to augment the benefits of other treatments without causing these severe complications. Very low doses of corticosteroids may be helpful as well.

Corticosteroids can also be injected directly into the affected joints for fast, short-term relief, but they can actually contribute to long-term damage. Because the pain is gone, you may be deceived into feeling as though nothing is wrong, especially with frequent injections. Overusing the joint can hasten its destruction.[9]

Corticosteroids are highly effective drugs for suppressing the inflammatory symptoms of rheumatoid arthritis.

DMARDs: Deeper Treatments for Rheumatoid Arthritis

The NSAIDs and pain killers described above can be used for all types of arthritis. However, there are other medications used for autoimmune forms of arthritis such as rheumatoid arthritis.

The major class of these drugs is called *disease-modifying antirheumatic* drugs, or DMARDs. They have received this description because they seem to be able to slow down the progression of rheumatoid arthritis, rather than just treat symptoms (see the sidebar Getting to the Root of the Problem).

What Do DMARDs Do?

The DMARDs each function in its own way, but the end results are somewhat similar. For all DMARDs, weeks or months of treatment are required for benefits to develop.

Getting to the Root of the Problem

NSAIDs and some of the rheumatoid arthritis drugs relieve symptoms but do not change the overall progression of the disease. As an analogy, consider a house that is "suffering" from termites. You could delay the house falling down by removing heavy furniture, tiptoeing about, and putting large beams under the joists; however, none of these methods would do anything to stop the gradual destruction of your house. Eventually, the termites would cause enough irreversible damage, and your house would collapse.

These delaying tactics are like NSAIDs. They treat the symptoms, but they don't address the underlying cause.

In the case of the termites, a more definitive approach would be to hire an exterminator to kill them. In medical terms, this would be described as a "disease-modifying" treatment.

The DMARD drugs act more like this approach. They reach deeply into rheumatoid arthritis and affect it closer to its root.

Each is at least partially effective in about two-thirds of patients, and when one fails to work, another may succeed. Good results include not only reduction of pain and inflammation, but also an improvement in the laboratory signs of rheumatoid arthritis. Sometimes, a drug in this family can even produce a full or partial remission that lasts after the drug is stopped.

This collection of effects has led to an impression that DMARDs somehow reach deeper in rheumatoid arthritis and get closer to its root than other drugs. Unfortunately, all the drugs in this category (with the possible exception of the new drug Enbrel) reliably cause severe side effects. Because of this toxicity, doctors have traditionally taken a "pyramid" approach with rheumatoid arthritis patients. Physicians started with NSAIDs to help with the pain and inflammation and only progressed to successively stronger and more toxic medications when the basic treatments failed.

Over the last few years, however, research has found that severe joint damage occurs very early in rheumatoid arthritis. In one study, x rays showed that more than 70% of patients had joint erosion and narrowing within 3 years of being diagnosed.[10] Furthermore, more damage occurred in the first year after diagnosis than during the next 2 years. This evidence

DMARDs can sometimes produce a full or partial remission that lasts even after you stop taking the drug.

has caused many authorities to suggest early, aggressive treatment with disease-modifying drugs to prevent joint damage.[11]

This approach makes good sense. There are, however, two things wrong with the strategy. First, all the traditional DMARDs are quite toxic and frequently cause severe side effects. Second, there is no definitive evidence that this strategy really works.[12] At present, the belief that DMARDs can actually prevent joint destruction in rheumatoid arthritis is just a hope.

As you'll see in chapter 9, fish oil supplements can relieve symptoms of rheumatoid arthritis, but there is no evidence that they can retard the progression of the disease. In general, natural options for rheumatoid arthritis are not as effective as are those for osteoarthritis. However, a number of exciting new conventional treatments have recently become available. The remainder of this chapter introduces the most important conventional treatments for rheumatoid arthritis.

Types of DMARDS

The traditional disease-modifying drugs for rheumatoid arthritis include antimalarials, gold salts, D-penicillamine, and sulfasalazine. The cancer drug methotrexate has recently joined the list, along with cyclosporine and the new drug leflunomide (Arava).

Antimalarials

Like many other drugs used for rheumatoid arthritis, this class of drugs was first used for another illness, in this case malaria. No one knows why antimalarials are effective in

Traditional DMARDs are quite toxic and frequently cause severe side effects.

treating rheumatoid arthritis. The most commonly used antimalarial is hydroxychloroquine sulfate (Plaquenil). About 70% of rheumatoid arthritis patients respond to this drug, at least to some extent. Hydroxychloroquine's most feared risk is vision loss due to retinal injury. Serious retinal damage occurs in less than 1% of those who use it,[13] but blindness is a frightening possibility, and it sometimes occurs months after the drug is discontinued.

Gold Salts

Gold salts, whether taken by injection or orally, are one of the most effective but toxic treatments for rheumatoid arthritis. Various gold compounds, administered orally or by injection, can suppress synovial inflammation, bring about partial or full remission, and perhaps slow joint damage. However, disturbing side effects develop in about one-third of patients who take gold, including changes in taste sensation, intense skin rashes that can be dangerous, and severe inflammation of mucous membranes. Less common but even more serious toxic effects include bone marrow injury, liver toxicity, and kidney damage.

D-Penicillamine

D-penicillamine is another dual-use drug also employed to treat certain forms of metal poisoning. It is about as effective as gold injections; but because it causes a high rate of serious reactions (up to 50%), it is usually only tried when gold fails. Common problems include fever, rash, itching, nausea and stomach pain, loss of appetite, mouth ulcers, and altered taste sensation. Serious injury to the bone marrow or kidneys is not infrequent.

Sulfasalazine

Sulfasalazine (Azulfidine EN-tabs), long used for inflammatory bowel disease, was recently approved by the Food and Drug Administration for rheumatoid arthritis as well. Although usually less effective than gold or penicillamine, it is also less toxic. Nonetheless, it can cause nausea, vomiting, abdominal pain, dizziness, and oversensitivity to the sun. Most seriously, sulfasalazine can sometimes cause a dangerous drop in a type of white blood cell known as neutrophils. To ward against this reaction, white count must be checked frequently during treatment.

Methotrexate

Methotrexate (Rheumatrex) has become increasingly popular for rheumatoid arthritis. It is an immune suppressant first developed for cancer chemotherapy. It can also be used to treat rheumatoid arthritis, juvenile rheumatoid arthritis, and lupus. Methotrexate has recently begun to be classed as a potential disease-modifying drug for rheumatoid arthritis.[14] Methotrexate often leads to improvement in symptoms within a month.

However, it can cause a host of side effects, including loss of appetite, nausea and vomiting, intestinal ulceration and, in some cases, bone marrow suppression and severe liver damage. As with sulfasalazine, patients taking methotrexate must be monitored for white blood cell count during therapy. Other side effects include headache, fatigue, malaise, and inflammation of the mouth (*stomatitis*).[15]

Lung inflammation, one of the most unpredictable and potentially serious side effects of treatment with methotrexate, can occur at relatively low doses.[16] Symptoms include shortness of breath, cough, fatigue, and fever.[17] In addition to lung disease, methotrexate can cause an increased incidence of bronchitis and pneumonia.[18]

There is also concern that methotrexate might increase the risk of blood cancers such as leukemia and lymphoma.[19] Although the evidence is contradictory, one study concluded that the spontaneous remission of lymphomas in rheumatoid arthritis patients after methotrexate was stopped was reason enough to further investigate the drug's role in development of these cancers.[20]

Cyclosporine

Cyclosporine is often used to suppress the immune system following organ transplants. It also provides benefits in rheumatoid arthritis, inducing rapid improvement when taken in high doses and slower improvement at low doses. There is some suggestion that cyclosporine may actually be a disease-modifying drug that can delay the appearance of new joint erosion,[21] although this is far from proven. Unfortunately, cyclosporine can cause numerous toxic effects, including seizures, inflammation of the brain, and kidney injury.

Leflunomide

The new kid on the immunosuppressant block is leflunomide, sold under the trade name Arava. Approved by the FDA in the fall of 1998, leflunomide is said to work by different mechanisms than most other immunosuppressing drugs. However, the exact mechanism is not certain. It appears to prevent more cells from being made in the synovial membrane by limiting cell division.[22]

Clinical trials of the drug demonstrated that it was able to relieve pain and swelling associated with rheumatoid arthritis, and it may slow damage to joints. Side effects seen most often in these trials included stomach upset, weight loss, rashes and other allergic reactions, and reversible hair loss. **Warning:** There are concerns, due to information from animal studies, that the drug may cause birth defects; it should not be used by pregnant women, or even by women not using reliable methods of birth control. Like most of the rheumatoid arthritis drugs, it may also be toxic to the liver, and should not be used by anyone with liver disease. Your doctor should check your liver enzymes periodically while you are using it.[23]

Antibiotic Therapy

As we discussed in chapter 3, one of the suspected causes of rheumatoid arthritis is infection by microorganisms such as bacteria, fungi, protozoa, or viruses. Studies in the early 1990s suggested that treatment with antibiotics known as tetracyclines might be beneficial for rheumatoid arthritis sufferers, and a number of clinical studies have confirmed this.

Minocycline, a member of this drug family, is the most commonly used for rheumatoid arthritis. This treatment has had a hard time gaining mainstream acceptance among doctors because the infection theory of rheumatoid arthritis is itself not widely accepted, and the supposed infectious organism has not been discovered.[24]

There is still debate about exactly how the drug works, or what percentage of people with rheumatoid arthritis it works for. Clinical studies have found that antibiotic treatment decreases both inflammation and the amount of rheumatoid factor in the blood. Proponents of the microorganism theory believe that it works as an antibiotic. However, there are other possible mechanisms as well. For example, minocycline appears to directly protect joints against damaging enzymes. It's possible that the fact that minocycline is an antibiotic too is a coincidence.

Side effects commonly seen with minocycline include stomach upset and dizziness—rather tame reactions, compared to some of the rheumatoid arthritis drugs' side effects.

A new drug, etanercept (Enbrel), approved in the fall of 1998, uses a unique approach to treat rheumatoid arthritis.

A New Therapeutic Approach: Etanercept (Enbrel)

This drug was approved in the fall of 1998. Its generic name is etanercept, and it's marketed as Enbrel. This drug uses a unique approach to treating rheumatoid arthritis. It contains a human protein that has been created using genetic engineering techniques. The protein resembles a receptor for a substance called "tumor necrosis factor" (TNF). TNF is one of the substances involved in creating the inflammation that leads to pain and eventual joint damage in rheumatoid arthritis. Etanercept essentially acts as a decoy, luring the TNF in close, and then latching on to it so that the TNF is unable to bind to the real receptors.

While some of the TNF may still find its way to the receptors, less of it does. This apparently limits the inflammation and may thereby slow down joint destruction.

Side effects seen with this drug were not serious. The most common side effect was of mild irritation on the skin at the point where the drug was injected. More patients in the therapeutic group had upper respiratory infections than in the placebo group, but these were reported as minor.

Because the drug is so new, little is known about the long-term effects. Long-term use studies are currently being conducted. Another unknown is how effective the drug would be for patients with a new onset of rheumatoid arthritis. Such studies are planned for the near future.

The drug is injected twice a week. At this point, it is quite expensive. Some insurance companies have reportedly been reluctant to pay for it, claiming it is an experimental treatment. However, now that FDA approval has been given, the manufacturer is apparently taking an active role in assisting patients with their insurance claims, and even has a certain amount of grant money available to cover the drug's cost for those who are truly unable to do so.

Other drugs that work in a similar fashion to etanercept are currently being researched.

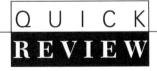

QUICK REVIEW

- The goals of conventional treatments for all types of arthritis focus on relieving pain, reducing inflammation, maintaining normal function, and preventing deformities.

- NSAIDs are the mainstay of treatment for osteoarthritis, and they are also used in the early stages of rheumatoid arthritis. However, they cause a high incidence of stomach distress and ulcers.

- There is also worrisome evidence that the NSAIDs may accelerate the progression of osteoarthritis. In contrast, many of the natural treatments described later in this book may actually slow the progression of osteoarthritis, although this is not known for certain.

- The most important drugs for rheumatoid arthritis are the disease-modifying antirheumatic drugs, the DMARDs. These offer the potential of slowing the progression of rheumatoid arthritis. However, most of them cause a high incidence of serious and often dangerous side effects. A new DMARD that has recently become available may be much safer.

Glucosamine Sulfate for Osteoarthritis

Right after turning 55, Helen had noticed the pain in her fingers. She was worried that this would interfere with her needlecraft, which was both a hobby and a source of income. She was soon diagnosed with osteoarthritis and given a prescription for Feldene.

The Feldene didn't help her arthritis, and she was afraid she might develop ulcers. In search of an alternative, she consulted Dr. Steven Bratman. He described the scientific evidence suggesting glucosamine as an effective treatment for osteoarthritis and recommended that she try 500 mg of glucosamine sulfate 3 times a day. He warned her that it might be as long as 4 weeks before she noticed any effects. Knowing from past experience that people often give up before the results develop, Dr. Bratman scheduled a return visit in a week.

Helen returned on schedule, ecstatic. She was pain free and could do her embroidery just like the old days. However, to her surprise, her doctor was not impressed. He told her that her results thus far were probably due to the power of suggestion alone, since none of the scientific studies had found a beneficial effect in such a short time. He asked her to come back the following week.

Sure enough, when she returned Helen complained that the glucosamine wasn't really working any better than Feldene. She was sad and depressed about the prospect that nothing would help her arthritis. Dr. Bratman explained again that her immediate benefit had likely been due to the placebo effect and reminded her that all the studies showed that it took time for glucosamine to work. He encouraged her to give it a fair trial.

When she came back in a month, she was smiling. "It's really working now," she said. When Dr. Bratman saw her after the second month of taking glucosamine, Helen reported that the pain relief was quite dramatic. She was doing her craft with no pain, and she was ecstatic that she could continue with needlework.

She continued taking glucosamine religiously for about 6 months, but then she ran out and forgot to get any more. After 3 months, her pain started to return. With this confirmation, Helen got back on her regimen of taking glucosamine and has been pain free ever since.

Of course, a story such as this one doesn't prove that glucosamine is effective. We need scientific research to know for sure. This chapter will present the evidence that for many people, glucosamine is effective for treating osteoarthritis, without any significant side effects.

A Brief History of Glucosamine

Glucosamine (glu-CO-sah-meen) was first isolated in 1878 from chitin, which makes up the hard covering, or exoskeleton, of such creatures as crustaceans, insects, and spiders. Chitin is still one of the primary sources of commercial glucosamine. Glucosamine is also found in the connective tissues of animals.

In the 1950s, laboratory studies reported that adding glucosamine to cultures of cartilage cells might stimulate an increased production of *proteoglycans* and *collagen,* which are used as "building blocks" for repair and manufacture of more cartilage cells. The use of glucosamine as a therapy for osteoarthritis was first reported in 1969 by German physicians, who used an injectable form of glucosamine.

Oral glucosamine has been approved in many European countries for treating osteoarthritis.

While some work research has continued with giving glucosamine by injection, there has also been a great deal of investigation into using glucosamine tablets. Oral glucosamine has been approved in many European countries for the treatment of osteoarthritis. American veterinarians have been using it to treat animals with arthritis, especially dogs and horses, with apparent success. Professional sports teams have also been using glucosamine. Between 30 and 50% of the Green Bay Packers are currently using the supplement, and trainers from other professional sports teams in the National Football League and National Basketball Association have begun providing their athletes with the supplement[1] in the as-yet undocumented hope that it will reduce the pain and disability of muscle and tendon injuries.

What Is Glucosamine?

Glucosamine is a molecule used by your body to make connective tissues. Because of its chemical structure, it can't exist by itself but must be bound to another substance. For this reason, when you find glucosamine in stores, it is usually as glucosamine sulfate. Sometimes you may also see glucosamine hydrochloride or acetylglucosamine. The sulfate form was the first to be commercially available in Europe and has been studied most extensively.

Glucosamine is one of the primary building blocks of the substances that make up both cartilage and synovial fluid, which lubricates the joints. Even though glucosamine is primarily produced in the body, a small amount may be supplied by the diet as well.

When you swallow a capsule containing glucosamine, approximately 90% is absorbed into your body. Some of it then enters the the joints, where it is incorporated into joint tissues.[2,3]

Your body uses glucosamine to make long-chain chemicals, called *glycosaminoglycans* (GAGs). These GAGs are then bound to protein cores to form proteoglycans. The end result resembles a pipe cleaner (on a microscopic scale)—the "wire" is made of the protein core, and the GAGs stick out all around. These molecules act like sponges to hold water, which makes up most of the weight of the cartilage, along with dissolved minerals and vitamins. The water acts like a shock absorber, helping connective tissue withstand forces that squeeze or stretch it.

It appears that taking supplemental glucosamine improves the health and quantity of these important parts of your joints, reducing pain and increasing mobility.

What Is the Scientific Evidence for Glucosamine?

A number of studies have provided evidence that glucosamine can relieve the pain caused by osteoarthritis. It appears to do so without significant side effects; and, unlike NSAIDs (see chapter 4), glucosamine appears to be generally healthy for cartilage rather than harmful. While the evidence at present is not definitive, it is impressive, and it has been enough to convince medical physicians throughout Europe, as well as veterinarians in the United States, to use glucosamine as a first-line treatment for arthritis. Some studies have compared glucosamine to placebo treatment, while others have compared it against standard arthritis drugs.

Glucosamine Versus Placebo

One of the best studies of glucosamine was a double-blind placebo-controlled study that involved 252 participants with osteoarthritis of the knee.[4] A total of 241 participants completed this 4-week trial. Of the 120 participants who received the glucosamine, 55% experienced a reduction in pain and stiffness (see figure 4). This was significantly better than the 38% rate of improvement among those who received the placebo.

Not only was glucosamine effective, it did not cause any significant side effects. To be precise, minor side effects, mostly upset stomach and allergy symptoms, were seen in about eight people taking glucosamine. However, similar side effects were seen in 13 people receiving placebo! When a treatment causes fewer side effects than placebo, it is reasonable to call it side-effect free for all practical purposes.

A number of studies have provided evidence that glucosamine can relieve the pain caused by osteoarthritis.

The major weakness of this trial was that it lasted only 4 weeks. For a chronic disease like osteoarthritis, you'd really like to have a study of at least 3 to 6 months' duration. But it still provides impressive evidence that glucosamine can be an effective treatment for osteoarthritis.

Similar results were seen in two other double-blind placebo-controlled studies, involving a total of 120 participants.[5,6]

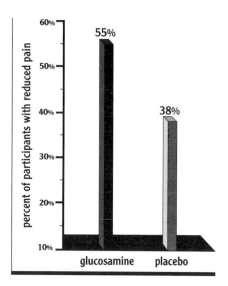

Figure 4. *Double-blind study shows that glucosamine can reduce the pain and stiffness of osteoarthritis* (Naack, 1994)

Glucosamine Versus Standard NSAIDs

A longer-term study compared the effects of glucosamine and the anti-inflammatory drug ibuprofen and found that they were equally effective. This double-blind comparison trial (meaning that it compared two treatments) involved 40 participants with osteoarthritis of the knee who attended a Portuguese clinic.[7] Over an 8-week period, 20 patients received 1,500 mg (500 mg 3 times a day) of glucosamine, while the other 20 received 1,200 mg of ibuprofen.

During the first 2 weeks of the study, ibuprofen appeared to be providing more pain relief than glucosamine. However, while the amount of relief gained from ibuprofen remained the same after that time, those in the glucosamine group continued to report gradual improvement throughout the study (see figure 5). It turned out to be a "tortoise and hare" situation—slow and steady won the race. By the end

Why the Knee?

You may wonder why all the studies described in this chapter use the knee joint. Indeed, earlier studies simply evaluated participants with osteoarthritis in any of the joints. However, it is hard to compare the osteoarthritis in one patient's shoulder with the severity of the disease in another person's finger joints! This difficulty made the results of such studies unreliable.

Researchers solved the problem by using a group of patients who all had problems with arthritis in the knee. Studying only one joint avoids trying to compare apples to oranges. Also, the knee joint was chosen because there is an easy way to rate the level of arthritis in the knee: see how far a person can walk without severe pain.

Scientific studies based on examining the level of arthritis in the knee joint have found that glucosamine can significantly relieve pain and improve mobility. This is good news for those suffering from arthritis in any joint.

of the 8 weeks, the patients taking glucosamine felt significantly better than the group taking ibuprofen.

Unfortunately, the dose of ibuprofen used in this study (1,200 mg) was half what is usually prescribed for the treatment of osteoarthritis. This means that the comparison wasn't really fair. Does glucosamine work as well as a full dose of ibuprofen? We don't really know.

This same study design was used again in the early 1990s in a study with 200 participants,[8] and more recently with a group of 178 individuals.[9] Again, the comparison dose of ibuprofen was on the low side, and these studies

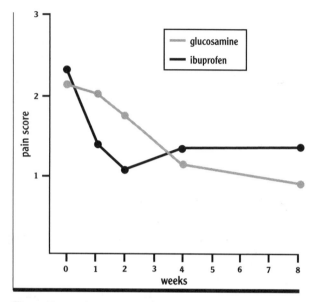

Figure 5. _Double-blind study shows that after 4 weeks of use, glucosamine provided greater pain relief than ibuprofen_ (Vaz, 1982)

lasted only 4 weeks. Similar results have been seen in other, smaller studies.[10–13]

One study did use full doses of an anti-inflammatory drug, and a stronger NSAID at that: piroxicam (Feldene). Results suggest that glucosamine can match the full benefits of appropriate drug treatment for osteoarthritis.

This study compared 1,500 mg of glucosamine to 20 mg of piroxicam per day. There were two other groups in the study as well: one that received placebo and another that received both piroxicam and glucosamine.[14,15,16] A total of 329 participants were enrolled, a sizable number that increases the study's validity. Another point in this study's favor was that the treatment lasted for 90 days.

Questionnaires given to the participants allowed the researchers to assign numeric scores representing their levels of pain and freedom of joint movement. At the end of 90 days, the participants completed the same questionnaires, and these were compared with the first set.

The results showed that glucosamine alone was at least as effective as piroxicam. Combining glucosamine and piroxicam didn't seem to add any extra benefit over using each treatment alone.

Again the glucosamine group had about the same number of reported side effects as the placebo group. This study had one more interesting feature. All treatment was stopped after 90 days, but patients were followed for an additional 60 days. Among patients given piroxicam, pain rapidly returned. However, the relief from glucosamine persisted. This seems to indicate that glucosamine is somehow doing more than just reducing symptoms of the disease.

All together, this was a very impressive study. It does have some problems, however. It has never been published at full length in a peer-reviewed scientific journal. The most complete description was only one page long, and it was given at a conference rather than published in a scientific journal.[17] Brief descriptions have been published in journals, but they disagree about some details![18,19]

Furthermore, numerous participants appear to have dropped out of the study before the end, somewhat decreasing the validity of the conclusions. These drawbacks are unfortunate, because this appears to be an impressive study with impressive results.

Putting All the Research Together

As of late 1998, a total of seven double-blind studies, involving 1,116 patients (see table 2), have been reported in English thoroughly enough to evaluate. Of these, three were placebo-controlled and four involved comparisons against medications. Although much still remains to be

Table 2. Summary of double-blind studies of glucosamine

Lead Author, Year	Number of participants	Length of study	Compared Against
Drovanti, 1980	80	30 days	Placebo
Pujalte, 1980	40	6 to 8 weeks	Placebo
Vaz, 1982	38	8 weeks	Ibuprofen, 1.2 g
Muller-Fassbender, 1994	199	4 weeks	Ibuprofen, 1.2 g
Noack, 1994	252	4 weeks	Placebo
Rovati, 1994, (Forster, 1996)	329	90 days, with a 60-day follow-up	Piroxicam, 20 mg, placebo, and combination
Qui, 1998	178	4 weeks	Ibuprofen, 1.2 g

discovered, this evidence does suggest that glucosamine provides relief for symptoms of osteoarthritis, apparently to the same extent as NSAID treatment, and with minimal side effects. The *Medical Letter on Drugs and Therapies* concluded that "glucosamine appears to be safe and might be effective for the treatment of osteoarthritis."[20]

There is as yet no evidence that glucosamine is useful for tendon and muscle problems, as sports teams seem to hope.

How Does Glucosamine Work?

We are not yet certain how glucosamine produces the results we have seen in clinical studies. However, we have strong suspicions that it works by helping joints resist damage.

One clue is that glucosamine does not appear to have any direct pain-relieving activity. It does appear to reduce inflammation, but only mildly, and by a different manner from the way NSAIDs work.[21] So if it isn't relieving pain and doesn't strongly reduce inflammation, it seems likely that it's working in some other manner altogether.

We do know that glucosamine can be used as raw material for making the substances involved in joints. Furthermore, evidence suggests that using glucosamine causes cartilage cells to manufacture more proteoglycans and collagen.[22,23,24] As described in chapter 1, the body fights osteoarthritis by creating new collagen and proteoglycans, but it can only keep up for so long. It may be that by helping the body rebuild cartilage, glucosamine can reduce the pain and stiffness of osteoarthritis. If this explanation is correct, there is a further aspect of glucosamine to consider. It may be that Holy Grail of arthritis treatments: a chondroprotective agent (an agent that stops arthritis from getting worse, or at least slows it down).

Can Glucosamine Stop or Slow the Progression of Osteoarthritis?

One of the most exciting possibilities with glucosamine, and some of the other osteoarthritis treatments described in this book, is the possibility that they can protect cartilage from damage, actually altering the course of the disease. Such a "chondroprotective agent" would be a major advance over all standard treatments.

As we have already said, glucosamine is both a raw material for the production of proteoglycans, and it also seems to be able to stimulate the production of new proteoglycans and collagen. This might give the body a boost in delaying the joint destruction of osteoarthritis.

Furthermore, recent evidence suggests that glucosamine can also inhibit the enzymes responsible for breaking down cartilage.[25] This would mean that it was working from both sides, as it were, to prevent the joints from deteriorating.

Unfortunately, we do not yet have any direct evidence that glucosamine really slows down osteoarthritis.[26] What we really need are long-term studies comparing the x-ray evidence of joint damage in two groups of subjects: the first given glucosamine, the second given placebo. Until such studies are performed, the promise of chondroprotection with glucosamine will remain only a promise.

As you will see in the next chapter, such studies have been reported for chondroitin sulfate, with positive results.

Dosages

The recommended dosage of oral glucosamine is 1,500 mg daily (500 mg 3 times a day with meals). In addition to 500-mg tablets and capsules, there are also some products

that offer other dosages, such as a 750-mg pill. You can take the 1,500 mg dosage by taking these pills twice a day. Glucosamine is also available in 1,500-mg packets that you can mix with juice or another beverage so that you only have to take it once a day. However you take it, taking glucosamine with meals helps prevent the possible side effect of an upset stomach.

Pain relief from glucosamine usually begins in 2 to 4 weeks and reaches maximum effect in 8 weeks.

Pain relief usually begins in 2 to 4 weeks and reaches maximum effect in 8 weeks. However, many people will not want to wait this long for pain relief. Research suggests that quicker results can be obtained by combining an NSAID along with glucosamine for the first 2 weeks to ensure prompt pain reduction until the glucosamine takes effect.[27]

Glucosamine is often sold in combination with chondroitin. However, although there are some theoretical reasons why chondroitin and glucosamine might work well when combined, we don't have any direct evidence that combination therapy is any better than glucosamine alone. Chondroitin by itself does appear to be effective, as described in chapter 6.

Safety Issues

Glucosamine appears to be extremely safe. It shows no toxicity even in extremely large doses;[28,29] and in the double-blind studies mentioned previously, it was not associated with any significant side effects.

One large study specifically looked at the safety of glucosamine. It involved 1,208 people who took glucosamine for almost 2 months. About 12% of the patients experienced side effects—mostly mild to moderate nausea or stomach upset. These symptoms are virtually inescapable, as they occur with placebo treatment as well.

The same study did suggest that patients on diuretics (drugs that promote the formation and release of urine) may need to take higher doses of glucosamine to get its full effect. There are no other known drug interactions.

However, maximum safe doses in young children, pregnant or nursing women, or those with severe liver or kidney disease has not been established. There are also concerns that glucosamine might be harmful for individuals with diabetes. It may raise blood sugar levels and also increase the risk of long-term diabetes side effects such as cataracts.

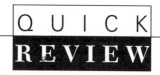

- Glucosamine is a substance used by your body to make connective tissues, such as cartilage and synovial tissue.

- In seven double-blind studies involving over 1,000 participants, glucosamine appears to provide symptomatic relief of osteoarthritis that was better than placebo and at least as effective as low-dose NSAID treatment.

- In test-tube studies, glucosamine has been found to stimulate the production of proteoglycans and collagen by cartilage cells. Glucosamine may also help protect cartilage from enzymes that break it down. This finding has led to the hope that glucosamine may be a chondroprotective agent (one that stops arthritis from getting worse or at least slows it down). Unfortunately, we don't as yet have any direct evidence for this exciting possibility.

- The recommended dose of glucosamine is 1,500 mg per day. This can be taken in divided doses or as one dose in a powdered form mixed with juice.

- Glucosamine causes few side effects, other than occasional mild stomach upset.

Chondroitin Sulfate for Osteoarthritis

Since osteoarthritis is a disease where cartilage is gradually damaged, a simplistic approach to treating it might involve gnawing the ends of bones, thereby ingesting cartilage or its constituents in the hope of strengthening and nourishing joint tissue. Although it's hard to believe that such an approach could really work, recent evidence suggests that one of the main ingredients of cartilage—chondroitin sulfate—not only reduces the symptoms of arthritis, but may slow the progression of the disease as well.

Chondroitin sulfate (kon-DROIT-uhn) is widely used in Europe for the treatment of arthritis—so widely, in fact, that in a recent editorial in the prestigious *Journal of Rheumatology,* chondroitin sulfate and its chemical cousins were described as "some of the most widely used therapies in osteoarthritis."[1] However, in Europe chondroitin sulfate is primarily used in a form that can be injected straight into arthritic joints. Injectable chondroitin sulfate is not widely available in the United States, but oral chondroitin sulfate has recently become extremely popular as a form of self-treatment for arthritis.

Reasonably good evidence suggests that chondroitin sulfate can significantly reduce the pain experienced with osteoarthritis.

There is now reasonably good evidence that chondroitin, like glucosamine, can significantly reduce the pain experienced with osteoarthritis. Furthermore, recent studies suggest that chondroitin can slow the usual progressive worsening of osteoarthritis. Remember, this same benefit has been proposed for glucosamine too. However, with glucosamine, this exciting possibility is mostly hypothetical. For chondroitin, there is actually some direct evidence to turn to.

What Is Chondroitin?

Chondroitin is one of a family of natural substances known as glycosaminoglycans (GAGs). It is composed of long chains that alternate two molecules: *galactosamine* and *glucuronic acid*. Galactosamine has the same chemical structure as glucosamine, but it has a slightly different three-dimensional shape. Like glucosamine, chondroitin is a molecule that can't exist alone. It must be paired with something—often sulfate.

The Controversy:
Is Oral Chondroitin Sulfate Absorbable?

Chondroitin sulfate became popular in the United States after the publication of Jason Theodosakis's *The Arthritis Cure,* which recommends combining it with glucosamine sulfate. Although there is considerable evidence supporting the use of injectable chondroitin sulfate, until recently there was little evidence that oral chondroitin sulfate worked. Indeed, many experts have gone on record stating that oral chondroitin sulfate cannot possibly work because it is too big a molecule to be absorbed. At best, they proposed, it is broken down into other substances (such as glucosamine) which then provide benefits.

Indeed, chondroitin sulfate is such a large molecule that at first glance it seems unlikely that it could be absorbed through the gut wall. In general, the gut cannot be penetrated by such enormous chemical structures. For example, cellulose is similar to chondroitin in many ways, and it simply passes through the digestive tract as dietary fiber. This opinion was bolstered by a small 1992 study that found that oral use of chondroitin sulfate did not raise blood levels of the substance.[2]

Direct evidence suggests that chondroitin can slow the usual progressive worsening of osteoarthritis.

However, more recent evidence suggests that chondroitin sulfate actually can be absorbed.[3,4] How such a molecule makes its way into the body is unclear, but apparently, it does. More important, we do have good evidence that when you take chondroitin, your arthritis symptoms will decrease.

What Is the Scientific Evidence for Chondroitin?

Until recently, the evidence for oral chondroitin sulfate was very weak. However, in 1998, the journal *Osteoarthritis and Cartilage* published a supplement devoted to updating the science on this supplement.[5] Three double-blind placebo-controlled studies were reported that provide evidence that chondroitin sulfate is an effective treatment for arthritis.

One of these was a 6-month double-blind placebo-controlled study that followed 85 participants with osteoarthritis of the knee.[6] In this study, participants received 400 mg of chondroitin sulfate twice a day or an identical-appearing placebo. Researchers evaluated improvement in arthritis symptoms by recording the level of pain as judged subjectively by the patient, the time it took to walk about 22 yards on flat ground, and the overall effectiveness of the treatment as rated by physicians and participants.

The results showed that after 1 month of treatment, there was a 23% decrease in joint pain in the chondroitin sulfate group versus only a 12% decrease in the placebo group (see figure 6). By 6 months there was a 43% improvement in the chondroitin sulfate group versus only a 3% improvement in the placebo group (the placebo effect sometimes wears off after a while). Walking speed did not improve over the 6 months with chondroitin sulfate (it stayed the same), while in the placebo group walking speed gradually and steadily declined. Finally, physicians rated the improvement as "good" or "very good" in 69% of those taking chondroitin sulfate but in only 32% of those taking placebo.

This was a reasonably long-term study that involved enough participants to be meaningful. However, another study lasted even longer, a full year, but it enrolled only 42 participants.[7] Again, the results showed that chondroitin sulfate produced tangible benefits as compared to placebo, with the differences generally increasing steadily over the entire year.

Another study was larger than either of these two, enrolling 127 participants, but it lasted for only 3 months.[8] Again, the results were positive.

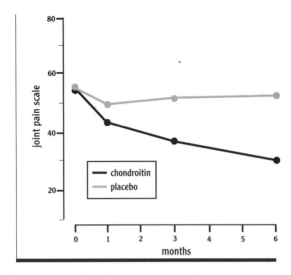

Figure 6. *Double-blind study showed chondroitin can decrease joint pain* (Busci and Poór, 1998)

Finally, an earlier study found that the benefits of chondroitin sulfate, like glucosamine sulfate, persist for months after treatment is stopped.[9] This study compared chondroitin sulfate to the drug diclofenac sodium (Voltaren). Two previous controlled studies also compared chondroitin sulfate to NSAIDs.[10,11] All together, six controlled trials have been performed in humans, involving a total of over 450 participants.

Can Chondroitin Sulfate Slow the Progression of Osteoarthritis?

The year-long study of chondroitin described earlier identified something quite remarkable beyond a reduction in pain and improvement in mobility: actual protection of the joints from damage.[12] Using x rays to assess the level of joint damage, researchers found that the severity of joint destruction gradually increased in individuals given placebo. However, among those taking chondroitin sulfate, no worsening of the joints was seen.

In other words, chondroitin sulfate seems to be able to slow the progression of osteoarthritis. This may be evidence of the long-sought-after chondroprotective treatment (a treatment that prevents arthritis from worsening) previously described for glucosamine sulfate. In this case, there seems to be some direct evidence, not just a hope.

X-ray evidence suggests that chondroitin sulfate actually protects joints from destruction.

No conventional treatment for osteoarthritis protects joints, and as described in chapter 4, some may actually harm joints in the long term. If confirmed by other studies, this finding may make chondroitin sulfate a distinctly superior treatment to NSAIDs or other conventional medications. Unfortunately, the small size of this study makes its evidence for cartilage protection less than conclusive.

A longer and larger double-blind placebo-controlled trial also looked at the progression of osteoarthritis by evaluating x rays of joints.[13] A total of 119 participants were enrolled in this study, which lasted a full 3 years. Thirty-four of the participants received 1,200 mg of chondroitin sulfate per day; the rest received placebo. Over the course of the study, researchers took x rays to determine how many joints had progressed to a severe stage of erosion.

During the 3 years of the study, only 8.8% of those who took chondroitin sulfate developed erosive joints. In comparison, almost 30% of those who took placebo progressed to this extent (see figure 7). This difference appears to be quite large. Unfortunately, the report did not state whether it was statistically significant, and it isn't

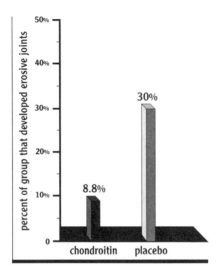

Figure 7. *Double-blind study shows that chondroitin seems to protect joints from erosion* (Verbruggen, Goemaere, and Veys, 1998)

possible for someone who reads the study to determine this crucial distinction from the information provided.

Additional evidence comes from animal studies. The effect of both oral and injected chondroitin sulfate was assessed in rabbits in which cartilage damage had been induced in one knee by the injection of an enzyme.[14] After 84 days of treatment in the animals who had been given chondroitin sulfate, the damaged knee had significantly more cartilage left than the knees of the untreated animals. Giving chondroitin sulfate by mouth was as effective as giving it through an injection.

Putting all this information together, it does appear that chondroitin sulfate can actually slow down the progress of osteoarthritis by protecting joints from damage. However, more studies are needed to confirm this very exciting potential benefit. Furthermore, none of this work demonstrates any power to reverse the disease by rebuilding the cartilage. Chondroitin sulfate may simply stop further destruction from occurring.

How Does Chondroitin Work?

At its most basic level, supplemental chondroitin sulfate may help cartilage by providing the body with the building blocks it needs to repair itself. Chondroitin sulfate is also believed to inhibit the activity of enzymes that break down cartilage. With less breakdown, there is a better balance between the constant breakdown and the building of new cartilage materials.[15]

Chondroitin sulfate is believed to inhibit the activity of enzymes that break down cartilage.

Additionally, chondroitin might act by increasing the amount of a beneficial substance named hyaluronic acid.[16] In Europe, hyaluronic acid is injected directly into joints and is another candidate for chondroprotective treatment. One study suggests that oral chondroitin can increase the amount of hyaluronic acid in the joints.[17]

Like glucosamine, chondroitin sulfate also appears to produce mild anti-inflammatory effects.[18] However, these are different from the type produced by NSAIDs. (To be technical, instead of affecting prostaglandins, chondroitin seems to inhibit the migration of inflammatory cells.)

Glucosamine, Chondroitin, or Both?

Since the publication of *The Arthritis Cure,* products containing a combination of glucosamine sulfate and chondroitin sulfate have become popular. Indeed, products containing just chondroitin sulfate are actually hard to find. The same combination is widely used in the veterinary world, where there is considerable evidence that the combination products are effective.[19] Unfortunately, no studies have been designed to determine whether the combination is more effective than either treatment alone. Nonetheless, there is some reason to believe that chondroitin sulfate and glucosamine sulfate might function synergistically.

As mentioned in chapter 5, glucosamine sulfate appears to stimulate cartilage cells to produce more of the building blocks of healthy joints. Chondroitin sulfate, as just described, may work in a complementary manner by inhibiting the enzymes that break down cartilage. It may therefore be reasonable to combine the two to achieve greater benefits.

However, as described in the last chapter, glucosamine sulfate may also inhibit those enzymes, and chondroitin itself is a building block of cartilage. In any case, we really need direct studies to know whether it is worth paying extra for the combination treatment.

We also don't know if one is more effective than the other. The best course is probably first to try one, and then (if you don't get results), try the other. If neither works, you might try the combination.

Dosage

Chondroitin sulfate is sold in 400-mg capsules. In most clinical studies, the dosage used was 800 to 1,200 mg daily.

Packets containing 1,200 mg of chondroitin sulfate have been developed for people to take as a convenient single daily dose, usually taken mixed with juice. One of the studies discussed above compared this new form of chondroitin sulfate with the same total dose taken in 3 separate pills and found equivalent benefits.[20] Enteric-coated capsules (designed to bypass the stomach and open up in the intestines) do not appear to be useful, as they reduce absorption.[21]

Glucosamine Sulfate and Chondroitin Sulfate: To Combine or Not to Combine?

Although we don't know whether combining chondroitin sulfate and glucosamine sulfate really works better than taking one of them alone, the combination certainly appears to be effective. Studies in animals have found a definite beneficial effect, and the treatment is widely accepted by veterinarians.[22,23] It seems to work in people, too.

Edward had just turned 50. One day while skiing—a sport he loved—he noticed a pain in his knee. He enjoyed his days hitting the slopes and didn't like the idea that he was getting "old" so soon. He tried taking an NSAID, but it upset his stomach too much. At one point he was afraid that he was getting an ulcer.

Chondroitin sulfate is more expensive than glucosamine sulfate. A year's supply costs almost $800, compared to $250 to $450 for glucosamine sulfate. On the plus side, only chondroitin sulfate has direct evidence that it slows osteoarthritis. The combination treatment costs even more—about $1,000 for the year's supply—which makes one wish a good study would come out telling us whether you really need to take both at once, or whether either one would do just as well.

Safety Issues

Chondroitin sulfate has not been associated with any serious adverse effects. This is not surprising, considering that taking it by mouth is essentially no different than chewing on gristle. Subjects in clinical trials have found mild digestive system distress to be the only real complaint.

A friend recommended a product that contained both chondroitin sulfate and glucosamine sulfate, which Ed began taking at the recommended dosage of 1,200 mg of chondroitin sulfate and 1,500 mg of glucosamine sulfate per day. It took 6 weeks before he noticed any pain relief, but he was very motivated and kept taking it. He is once again enjoying skiing.

However, we don't know whether he really needed to pay the extra premium to buy a combination of chondroitin sulfate and glucosamine sulfate. From the available scientific evidence, we simply don't know if the combination treatment is any more effective than each individual constituent.

Although it does not seem likely that any problem should develop, chondroitin's safety has not been proven in young children, pregnant or nursing women, or those with severe liver or kidney disease.

Other Substances Like Chondroitin That Have Been Used for Osteoarthritis

Besides chondroitin sulfate, there are other GAGs that have been suggested as treatments for osteoarthritis. These include chitin, gelatin, and some sea animals.

Chitin

Chitin is composed of long, unbranched chains of a chemical called N-acetylglucosamine (NAG). NAG is the most abundant GAG in nature. It is a natural component of the

The Problem with Testimonials

As we wrote this in 1998, we ran across a letter in the *Seattle Times*.[24] This letter cites several anecdotal claims of the relief of osteoarthritis symptoms by taking a grocery store pectin product.

Pectin is a polysaccharide found in high concentration in apples, similar in structure to GAGs, and widely used in making jams and jellies. To my knowledge there are no studies of the use of this substance to treat osteoarthritis. However, the text of the letter provides an interesting insight into how anecdotes of potential remedies are spread.

"You recently expressed surprise that Certo—a pectin-containing solution used for making jams and jellies—has been used for arthritis since the 1970s.

"Back in 1945, my 65-year-old grandmother suffered from arthritic knees—almost surely osteoarthritis. A friend told her

shells of insects and crustaceans and is the raw material from which glucosamine sulfate is produced. However, there simply hasn't yet been any significant level of investigation into whether NAG itself is effective for osteoarthritis or how it compares with chondroitin sulfate.

Gelatin

Gelatin was probably the first substance proposed as a treatment for arthritis, on the theory that if you eat material similar to what is in joints, it will make your joints healthier. Gelatin is derived from collagen, the protein component of cartilage. It is obtained by boiling skin, tendons, ligaments,

about the benefits of Certo in fruit juice; she was pain free within a few weeks.

"I ruled out the placebo effect because during a 2-week vacation she had no access to Certo and was a wreck when she returned. Back to taking Certo, she was fine in 2 weeks." (Authors' note: this does not rule out the placebo effect at all.)

"A few years ago, I noticed persistent pain in my thumbs, shoulders, wrists, and elbows. A nurse practitioner diagnosed osteoarthritis and offered anti-inflammatory pills.

"I tried a tablespoon of Certo mixed with fruit juice (mostly grape) at breakfast and bedtime. Within a couple of weeks my symptoms disappeared—only to reappear with a vengeance when I stopped Certo, and vanish when I returned to Certo."

Unfortunately, testimonials like this are a dime a dozen in medicine. They don't prove anything at all, and almost never pan out when they are scientifically evaluated.

and bone of cows, pigs, and horses in water. However, there is no scientific evidence for the use of gelatin in arthritis.

From the Sea

The search for natural substances to prevent or reverse the effects of osteoarthritis has led people to try many other substances that are related to cartilage or that participate in its creation by the body. Two of the most popular extracts in the natural foods market have been the green-lipped mussel and the sea cucumber.

The New Zealand green-lipped, or Perna, mussel, *Perna canaliculus,* has been marketed since the 1960s as a natural treatment for arthritis. However, there is no direct evidence that this extract works.

Despite its vegetable-like name, the sea cucumber (*Pseudocolochirus axiologus*), is a sea animal related to starfish and sea urchins. It has served as a food staple in southeast Asian cultures and has been used in traditional Chinese medicine as a treatment for a variety of conditions. Sea cucumbers are rich in GAGs, including chondroitin sulfate. However, once more, there have not been any adequate studies of this proposed arthritis treatment.

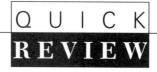

QUICK REVIEW

- A growing body of double-blind studies suggests that chondroitin, a naturally occurring component of cartilage, may be an effective treatment for osteoarthritis.

- The typical dose is 800 to 1,200 mg of chondroitin sulfate daily.

- Besides reducing pain, evidence suggests that chondroitin may protect cartilage from destruction, thereby slowing the progression of osteoarthritis.

- Chondroitin may also function well in combination with glucosamine, although this too has not been proven.

S-Adenosylmethionine (SAMe) for Osteoarthritis

S -adenosylmethionine, or SAMe for short (sometimes known by the name SAM), appears to be a safe and effective treatment for osteoarthritis. SAMe may also be a chondroprotective substance (one that slows the progression of osteoarthritis). However, despite all its promise, there is one severe problem with SAMe: its price. This is a very expensive supplement.

What Is SAMe?

SAMe (pronounced "sam-ee") is one of the most fundamental molecules in the human body. It is closely related to the substance ATP (adenosine tri-phosphate), the molecule that stores the energy derived from the food we eat and the oxygen we breathe. The body uses ATP as a kind of "energy currency" to deliver energy to the specific sites in the cells where work must be done. Every action in the body that requires an input of energy depends on ATP, including nerve impulses, muscle contractions, and tissue building.

ATP combines with the amino acid methionine to form another molecule, S-adenosylmethionine (SAMe). SAMe is formed in every cell of the body, and it is essential for many of the biochemical reactions our lives depend on.[1]

Also known as ademetionine, SAMe was first discovered by Italian chemists in 1952.

SAMe appears to be a safe and effective treatment for treating osteoarthritis.

SAMe is a very unstable molecule—it tends to break apart quickly after it is created. It was not until the mid-1970s that chemists were able to manufacture it in a way that kept it intact, making it available in forms suitable for clinical investigations.

Because Italian researchers were the first to discover SAMe's role in treating osteoarthritis, most of the subsequent research into SAMe has been performed in Italy. However, unlike much of the research on natural substances done outside the United States, all of this work is accessible to American doctors. The *American Journal of Medicine,* in a supplement devoted entirely to the research on SAMe, published reports of eight controlled comparative studies, four uncontrolled studies, and a good review of the entire body of research.[2] This research strongly suggests that SAMe is an effective treatment for osteoarthritis.

What Is the Scientific Evidence for SAMe?

SAMe has been the subject of many studies. The most practical ones fall into one of three categories: double-blind placebo-controlled studies, double-blind comparative studies, and open studies.

The best of these is the double-blind placebo-controlled study. In such studies, some participants are given the real treatment and others are given a phony treatment, but neither doctors nor participants know which is which. When properly performed, this type of study completely eliminates the power of suggestion. There have been at least two double-blind placebo-controlled studies of SAMe involving a total of over 700 people.

The second best type of study is also double-blind, but it compares a new treatment against another one that is already known to be effective. This type of study isn't as reliable as a placebo-controlled study, but it still provides meaningful information. About 500 people have participated in these studies, sometimes called double-blind comparative trials.

The least meaningful form of study is called an open or uncontrolled trial. Such studies are not blinded, meaning nothing is hidden from doctors or participants, and there is no placebo group. Participants are simply given a treatment, and researchers record what happens. In such studies, it isn't possible to determine which effects are due to the treatment itself and which are due to the placebo effect. The main use of open studies is to look for severe adverse effects of a treatment. For this reason, they are sometimes called "drug-monitoring studies." A grand total of over 20,000 people have been followed in open trials of SAMe, giving us considerable evidence for the safety of this treatment.

Putting the information together, these studies tell us two things. First, they provide substantial evidence that SAMe is an effective treatment for osteoarthritis, about as effective as standard NSAIDs. Second, it does not cause any serious side effects. However, more research needs to be done, primarily because most of the studies performed to date were quite short.

Double-Blind Placebo-Controlled Studies

One of the best studies of SAMe combines features of placebo-controlled and comparative studies. The results

Accidental Discoveries

Not all side effects are bad. Sometimes a treatment being studied for a particular problem has been found to have a positive "side effect" that may make it useful for a separate and perhaps totally unrelated problem. The famous pharmacologist from the Philadelphia College of Pharmacy and Science, Dr. G. Victor Rossi, has always been fond of saying, "Today's side effects are tomorrow's therapy."

For example, researchers investigating iproniazid, an early treatment for tuberculosis, were surprised by how much happier some of their participants became. They wondered if participants were just pleased to be getting over their TB or whether more was going on behind the scenes. A closer look revealed that iproniazid was successfully treating depression in those patients who had become depressed by their disease. The whole category of antidepressant drugs began with this accidental discovery.

There are many more examples. Antipsychotic drugs came out of research into antihistamines, and a treatment pre-

showed that SAMe was clearly more effective than placebo and produced equivalent benefits to the drug naproxen, with fewer side effects.

This double-blind placebo-controlled trial enrolled 734 participants and followed them for 4 weeks.[3] Over this period, 235 of the participants received 1,200 mg of SAMe per day; a similar number took either a placebo or 750 mg daily of the standard drug naproxen. The majority of these participants had experienced moderate symptoms

scribed for high blood pressure has proved useful for symptoms related to enlargement of the prostate.

The discovery that SAMe provided relief from the pain of osteoarthritis was one of these serendipitous findings, unrelated to the original research question. SAMe was first investigated as an antidepressant drug. However, Italian researchers noticed that depressed participants who also happened to have osteoarthritis reported that they had fewer symptoms of their joint disease.

If you are less depressed, you hurt less, so at first researchers attributed the reported improvements to this effect. But it seemed to be more than that. Eventually, clinical trials were conducted specifically to see whether SAMe can help osteoarthritis. At this point, the evidence is probably better for osteoarthritis than for depression.

SAMe also has other positive side effects. It seems to protect both the liver and the stomach from injury. If only all side effects were this good!

of osteoarthritis of either the knee or the hip for an average of 6 years.

The dosage of naproxen used in this study falls toward the lower end of the dosage range recommended for the treatment of arthritis, which is 500 to 1,500 mg per day. Nonetheless, it was high enough to produce some benefits.

Participants were examined at the beginning of the study, after 2 weeks, and again at 4 weeks. Evaluations of the success of treatment were based on the participants' reports of their level of pain as well as their capacity to perform normal activities.

The results indicate that SAMe provided as much pain-relieving effect as naproxen and that both treatments

Research strongly suggests that SAMe is an effective treatment for osteoarthritis.

were significantly better than placebo. However, differences did exist between the two treatments. Naproxen worked more quickly, producing readily apparent benefits at the 2-week follow-up, whereas the full effect of SAMe was not apparent until 4 weeks. By the end of the study, both treatments were producing the same level of benefit. We do not know whether further improvement would have been seen in the SAMe group had the study continued longer, or whether the benefits would have faded away.

Another difference was that naproxen caused more side effects than SAMe, primarily digestive distress.

Putting all this information together, it is safe to say that SAMe is more effective than placebo and equally effective as 750 mg a day of naproxen while causing fewer side effects. However, SAMe takes longer to work than naproxen, and we don't know whether higher dosages of naproxen, such as are commonly used for osteoarthritis, might be more effective.

There has only been one other double-blind placebo-controlled study of SAMe, a 4-week trial of about 80 people. For technical reasons, however, its results are not meaningful.[4] (The problem was that the group of participants given SAMe did not have the same level of symptoms as the placebo group. This makes comparing the results like comparing apples and oranges.)

Comparative Studies

Besides these two double-blind placebo-controlled studies, only one of which was meaningful, there have been several comparative studies as well. As we mentioned above, a comparative study compares the action of a new treatment to an established treatment. It is not as reliable as a placebo-controlled study, but it does supply meaningful information.

In the most recent of the double-blind comparative trials, SAMe was found to be equally effective as the drug piroxicam (Feldene).[5] This study was the longest of the controlled studies on SAMe performed to date, and it is also notable for using a full dosage of the anti-inflammatory drug (20 mg) instead of a low dosage. A total of 45 participants were treated for 84 days and then followed for an additional 56 days after treatment was stopped. The effectiveness of the treatments were measured by participants' reports regarding their level of pain and stiffness and by the researchers' observations of symptoms such as range of motion of the affected joint and the degree of swelling present.

The results showed that SAMe and piroxicam produced quite similar benefits. Both treatments reduced pain significantly within the first 4 weeks but required 8 weeks to reduce stiffness. SAMe took longer to improve range of motion than piroxicam, but ultimately it was just as effective for this symptom. Both treatments reduced the amount of fluid that had collected in the knee joint.

Then, at the end of 84 days, all participants were transferred to placebo (without their knowledge) for an additional 4 weeks. During that time, the participants treated with SAMe maintained their clinical improvement longer than those treated with piroxicam. As described in chapter 5, this same kind of effect has been seen with glucosamine.

It is one of the findings that has raised hopes that SAMe can alter the fundamental course of osteoarthritis. For if SAMe can produce results that last long after the treatment has washed out of the blood, it must be actually improving the health of the joint in some way.

Several other studies, involving a total of about 450 people, have compared SAMe to anti-inflammatory drugs, primarily ibuprofen (Advil).[6–10] All of them found SAMe to be equally effective to NSAID drugs. However, in most cases, the dosage of anti-inflammatory used was on the low side.

Open Studies

There have also been open studies of SAMe. As mentioned earlier in this chapter, in open studies, both the participants and the doctors evaluating them know everything that is going on, and there is no placebo group. Such studies do not eliminate the power of suggestion. For this reason, they are more useful for providing information about side effects and safety of long-term use than about effectiveness.

The results of two open studies suggest that SAMe produces few side effects, and those that do occur disappear after a while. One of these studies was impressive for its size (over 20,000 participants) and the other for its length (2 years). That such studies could even be performed is a testament to SAMe's popularity in Europe.

The first open study enrolled more than 20,000 participants and followed them for 56 days as they took SAMe.[11] None of these participants was allowed to take pain-relievers or other drugs for their arthritic symptoms. The effect of treatment was rated as "very good" or "good" in 71% of the cases, as "moderate" in 21%, and as "poor" in 9%. However, as stated earlier, it is impossible to tell how much of this effect was due to the power of suggestion.

More important, the large majority tolerated SAMe treatment quite well. Only 5% of the participants discontinued the treatment early because of unpleasant side effects (primarily mild digestive distress), and 2.3% quit because they didn't perceive any success.

The other open study enrolled 108 participants and followed them for 2 years while they took SAMe.[12] Again, most participants had good results, and very few side effects were reported. In fact, of the 108 participants who started the study, 106 completed the first year of the study, and only 11 had dropped out by the end of the study. This is a very low dropout rate. Side effects that did occur tended to decrease with time, and during the last 6 months of the study, no side effects were reported at all. Laboratory measurements conducted over the course of the study found no health problems caused by SAMe.

SAMe appears to be a very safe treatment.

The bottom line is that SAMe appears to be a very safe treatment.

How Does SAMe Work in Osteoarthritis?

We don't know exactly how SAMe works in osteoarthritis, but we do have some ideas. According to animal studies, SAMe does seem to have some direct anti-inflammatory and pain-relieving effects.[13] However, SAMe does not appear to work in the same way as NSAIDs (specifically, it does not alter prostaglandin levels).

Perhaps more important, SAMe seems to have positive effects on cartilage cells. Evidence derived from test tube studies[14] suggests that SAMe stimulates those cells to produce more proteoglycans, which, as we saw in chapter 1, are important substances for maintaining healthy cartilage. Furthermore, when people are given SAMe orally, blood levels of proteoglycans increase.[15] Thus SAMe may improve arthritis symptoms by actually making joints healthier, rather than just relieving pain and reducing inflammation.

Is SAMe a Chondroprotective Agent?

Three types of evidence suggest that SAMe may be a chondroprotective agent, a substance that slows the progression of osteoarthritis. First, as noted earlier, SAMe's benefits have been found to continue for months after treatment is stopped. Second, SAMe has been found to increase production of proteoglycans, substances used to build and repair cartilage. Finally, evidence from a study in animals gives us additional reason for enthusiasm. It suggests that SAMe may help protect joints from developing arthritis.

SAMe seems to have positive effects on cartilage cells.

In this study, rabbits were given a surgical treatment that tends to cause arthritis.[16] Then some were given SAMe, while others were not. Treated rabbits showed significant protection against the development of arthritis. Their cartilage was thicker, it had more cartilage cells, and proteoglycan levels were also higher. This is pretty good evidence that SAMe can protect and rebuild cartilage in a living animal.

Still, in order to know whether SAMe slows down the progression of normal osteoarthritis in people, we would need long-term controlled studies that specifically look for the progression of arthritis. Unfortunately, no study of this type has yet been reported.

Dosage

The usual dosage of SAMe is 400 mg 3 times a day until symptoms improve. Then, if relief from your symptoms is achieved, it is quite possible that as little as 200 mg per day will keep symptoms under control. Keep in mind that in the studies mentioned above, it took as long as a month for the full effect of SAMe to be felt.

Some people experience digestive distress when they first take SAMe. If this happens to you, starting with a lower dosage and working up gradually should take care of it.

The full effects of SAMe may take as long as a month to be felt.

Safety Issues

SAMe seems to be a very safe treatment. In the open study of over 20,000 people, no serious adverse side effects could be attributed to SAMe, although mild stomach distress occurred occasionally. In the 2-year study of SAMe, side effects that did develop initially tended to go away over time.

SAMe also has some positive "side effects." Perhaps the most important is that SAMe appears to be effective as an antidepressant. Remember that its use in arthritis was originally a "side effect" of its use in depression. Since people with pain and impaired function are more likely to be depressed, this could be a very much appreciated side effect for some people with osteoarthritis. (For more information on SAMe and its possible use in depression, see *The Natural Pharmacist Guide to St. John's Wort and Depression.*) However, don't combine SAMe with standard antidepressant drugs, as there is at least one report of a harmful interaction between them.[17]

> **Unlike NSAIDs, which can damage the stomach lining after extended use, SAMe seems to actually protect the lining of the stomach.**

Another potential beneficial side effect of SAMe is that, quite the opposite of NSAIDs, it seems to actually protect the lining of the stomach.[18,19] Studies suggest that it can counter the harmful effects of alcohol and aspirin. Since the major problem with NSAID drugs is that they frequently damage the stomach lining over time, this appears to be a major advantage with SAMe.

There is also some evidence that SAMe can protect the liver from damage caused by alcohol and other liver toxins.[20] With "side effects" like these, the term takes on a whole new meaning.

What Are the Drawbacks?

At this point, if you are suffering from arthritic pain, you might be thinking, "SAMe sounds pretty good. I think I'd like to try it. What are the drawbacks?"

Besides the minor side effects mentioned already, the major drawback to using SAMe is that it is incredibly expensive. A full dosage of 1,200 mg daily could cost hundreds of dollars a month.

If it gets to be more commonly used, the price may begin to come down. But at the present time, even if it is medically effective, SAMe is not cost-effective. If glucosamine sulfate is as medically effective, or even a little less effective than SAMe, then it would certainly be a much better choice from the point of view of price.

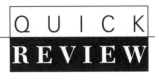

- Fairly strong evidence indicates that SAMe is a safe and effective treatment for osteoarthritis. However, it is very expensive.

- The benefits from using SAMe for osteoarthritis appear to last for months after treatment is stopped. Together with evidence from test tube and animal studies, this suggests that SAMe may be a chondroprotective treatment (one that slows progression of the disease).

- Start with 400 mg 3 times a day, and then taper down gradually when symptoms improve. As little as 200 mg per day might be sufficient to maintain improvement.

- Some people develop upset stomach from SAMe, but this usually goes away in time. If it is severe, try reducing the dosage and then increasing it gradually.

- SAMe is also believed to produce positive side effects, including fighting depression and protecting the stomach and liver from damage.

Herbs for Osteoarthritis

T he use of plants to treat illnesses and injuries has a very long history. The earliest human beings lived surrounded by plants that provided much of their food, fiber, and medicine. It is thought that human beings discovered the therapeutic benefits of plants through a process of trial and error. In whatever way human beings learned the healing powers of certain plants, there can be no doubt that their use has been long and pervasive.

Circumstantial evidence from the burial site of a Neanderthal man in the mountains of what is now northern Iraq suggests that early humans used some plants as herbal medicines that are still used today for this purpose.[1] Certainly, herbal medicines are the central ingredients in all traditional medicine systems around the world. The World Health Organization estimates that 75 to 80% of the world's population relies exclusively on plants and plant extracts for their primary health-care needs.[2,3]

Osteoarthritis has been a scourge of humanity for a long time, and it is not surprising that many herbs have been used in one way or another to treat it. Most of these herbs have not been investigated to the same extent as St. John's wort or ginkgo. Nonetheless, there is some research to cite. In this chapter, we'll look at a few of the herbs that possess at least a modest scientific basis.

Scientific Herbal Medicine: Phytotherapy

The role medicinal plants have played in the development of modern pharmacology might surprise you. Many drugs were originally derived from plants, including morphine, quinine, digitalis, pseudoephedrine (Sudafed), aspirin, guaifenesin (the expectorant in all cough syrups), and the anticancer agents vinblastine, vincristine, and taxol. Approximately three-fourths of these were originally investigated by the pharmaceutical companies because of their use in traditional medicine.

Archeological evidence suggests that Neanderthal man used some medicinal herbs we use today.

One of the earliest and most influential systematic treatises on the clinical uses of plants in Western civilization is the *Materia Medica,* written by Pedanius Dioscorides in the first century A.D. Dioscorides was an itinerant Greek physician who served in the Roman army of Nero's time. His text became the basis of the herbals of the Middle Ages, though a great deal of myth and superstition became attached to this body of knowledge.

As modern medicine developed, it became increasingly common to extract active ingredients from herbs and use them as drugs. Whole herbs, too, continued to be used as treatments, although they were regarded as less ideal. By about the time of World War II, most physicians in the United States had entirely lost interest in herbal medicine.

However, researchers in Germany and other European countries continued to investigate the use of herbal medications. Phytotherapy (from *phyto,* meaning plant)—a new and more scientific approach to herbal medicine—developed out of their efforts. The recent interest in herbs such as ginkgo and St. John's wort stems primarily from this European research.

Research has also focused on herbal remedies used to treat osteoarthritis. In this chapter we'll discuss the findings on the safety and effectiveness of plant medicines such as willow bark, devil's claw, boswellia, and a compound taken from hot peppers, capsaicin.

Willow Bark:
The Original Anti-Inflammatory

It all started with willow bark. Almost all the present-day drugs used for osteoarthritis owe their origin to this common plant. The bark of the willows *(Salix spp.),* poplars *(Populus spp.),* and other trees belonging to the willow family *(Salicaceae)* contains a chemical called salicin. Salicin is also found in the herb meadowsweet.

Willow bark has a long history in the treatment of gout and arthritis. Dioscorides recommended it, taken with wine and pepper, as a treatment for joint pain. In 1829, salicin was chemically extracted from willow and found to have medicinal properties. In 1835, a German chemist chemically altered salicin into salicylic acid and marketed it as an arthritis drug. For his source of salicin, he used the herb meadowsweet instead of willow bark. Because the Latin name for meadowsweet is *spirae,* he called this chemical spiric acid. Salicylic acid has anti-inflammatory, analgesic (pain-reducing), and antipyretic (fever-reducing) activities and is the prototype of all nonsteroidal anti-inflammatory drugs (NSAIDs) such as ibuprofen.

But salicylic acid is very irritating to the stomach. In fact, today it is often used to burn off warts. Felix Hoffman, a chemist in the Bayer division of the German chemical company I. G. Farben, sought to develop a less irritating form of the substance for his arthritic father.[4] In 1898, he chemically modified salicylic acid by combining it with acetic acid, turning it into acetyl–salicylic acid. Since it was a combination of acetic acid and spiric acid, he

Willow bark has a long history in the treatment of gout and arthritis.

named this product *aspirin,* and marketed it as the still-famous Bayer aspirin. Aspirin is much less irritating to the stomach than salicylic acid, although stomach problems are still the major side effect of this medication.

The herb that started it all, willow bark, is itself enjoying a comeback. Today, Germany's Commission E, a body charged with the task of regulating the use of herbal medicines, recognizes willow bark for the treatment of "feverish illnesses, rheumatic disorders and headaches," the same conditions for which aspirin is regularly prescribed.

Dosage

Commission E recommends a dosage of willow that will supply 60 to 120 mg of salicin daily. Willow bark is probably most effective when taken as a tea because not much salicin is absorbed from the powdered herb.[5]

Safety Issues

Interestingly, the salicin present in willow bark does not appear to be particularly irritating to the stomach.[6]

However, salicin is converted into salicylic acid once it is inside the body. It therefore has the potential to cause all the same effects as aspirin, including stomach ulcers, allergic reactions, and Reyes syndrome (a serious kidney disorder that can occur when children take aspirin). Willow bark is not recommended for young children or pregnant or nursing women.

Because of its salicin content, willow bark may interact with other anti-inflammatory drugs as well as anticoagulants, methotrexate, metoclopramide, phenytoin, probenecid, spironolactone, and valproate.

Devil's Claw:
A Promising African Herb

Devil's claw, *Harpagophytum procumbens*, is a plant native to the Kalahari Desert of South Africa and Namibia, where it is used as a fever reducer and analgesic. Its claw-like appearance is the source of its common name.

Devil's claw was introduced into European herbal medicine in 1953. Presently, the German Commission E monograph, an official report from the German equivalent of the U.S. Food and Drug Administration, suggests the herb can be used for "degenerative disorders of the locomotor system," meaning arthritis. More recently, the European Scientific Commission on Phytotherapy (ESCOP) reported that devil's claw is useful for arthritis and tendinitis.[7] Devil's claw has become a popular herbal treatment for arthritis of all kinds.

> **Devil's claw has become a popular herbal treatment for arthritis of all kinds.**

Devil's claw contains substances called iridoid gluco-sides, principally harpagoside, harpagide, and procum-bide. Devil's claw products are usually standardized on the basis of either their harpagoside or total iridoid glucoside content.

What Is the Scientific Evidence for Devil's Claw?

To date, three double-blind placebo-controlled studies in-volving devil's claw have been reported. Two examined participants with various forms of arthritis, while the other study looked at participants with low back pain.

The first study measured pain reduction in 50 volun-teers with arthritis. Half were given 800 mg of standardized devil's claw extract (containing 1.5% iridoid glucosides) 3 times daily over a period of 3 to 8 weeks, while the other half received placebo.[8] Compared with placebo, devil's claw produced a statistically significant reduction in the severity of pain. The author reported that meaningful improve-ments were seen more frequently in moderate cases than in severe ones.

The second double-blind placebo-controlled study in-volved 89 participants with "rheumatoid complaints" (an annoyingly vague term).[9] They received 670 mg of pow-dered herb (containing 3% iridoid glucosides) 3 times daily for 2 months. In order to evaluate the effects of the herb, researchers measured subjective pain scores as well as how far participants could bend at the waist. Both of these showed significant improvement when measured at 30 and at 60 days.

How Does Devil's Claw Work?

We don't know exactly how devil's claw helps in arthritis. However, animal studies suggest that, like NSAIDs, devil's claw has two effects: relieving pain and reducing inflammation.

Interestingly, devil's claw appears to affect inflammation by some mechanism that is very different from that of conventional anti-inflammatories. Those medications produce certain characteristic changes in the levels of prostaglandins and other chemicals that "mediate" or play a crucial role in inflammation. However, a 3-week study of 25 healthy volunteers given devil's claw found no change in the levels of these substances you would expect to see from treatment with a conventional NSAID medication.[10] It's possible that a whole new approach to anti-inflammatory treatment may emerge from studies of this interesting herb.

Dosage

The European Scientific Commission on Phytotherapy (ESCOP) monograph recommends a dose of 1 to 3 g of devil's claw root 3 times daily for the treatment of arthritis and tendinitis. If standardized to iridoid glucosides (2 to 3%) or harpagoside (1 to 2%), the dose should be lower, generally about 600 to 800 mg 3 times daily.

Based on animal studies indicating that stomach acid damages the constituents of devil's claw, some authors have suggested that the herb should be provided in a special form (enteric coated) that bypasses the stomach. However, there is no evidence yet that such a product would work better.

Safety Issues

Animal studies of devil's claw and its components have found a very low level of toxicity both short and long term.[11] With mice, doses as high as 7.5 g per kg were found to be harmless. Scaled upward, this corresponds to more than 100 times the suggested daily dose for people. In a 6-month drug-monitoring study of 630 participants with arthritis, no side effects were reported other than occasional mild digestive distress.[12]

NSAIDs can cause ulcers, presumably because they reduce the production of prostaglandins that protect the stomach from damage. Because devil's claw does not appear to affect prostaglandins, this same risk should not apply. Even so, for reasons that are not entirely clear, European herbalists often recommend against use of devil's claw by those with ulcers.

The safety of this herb for young children, pregnant or nursing women, or those with severe heart, liver, or kidney disease has not been established. There are no known drug interactions with devil's claw, although there are theoretical concerns that devil's claw might interfere with drugs used to prevent abnormal heart rhythms.

Boswellia: More Commonly Used for Rheumatoid Arthritis

In Ayurvedic medicine (the traditional medicine in India), a resinous gum extracted from the *Boswellia serrata* tree is used for osteoarthritis, rheumatoid arthritis, and similar conditions. Research suggests that the boswellic acids found in boswellia have anti-inflammatory effects. As with devil's claw, these effects appear to occur by a different route than that of other anti-inflammatory drugs. Although boswellia may have a role in osteoarthritis, most of the scientific investigation has focused on rheumatoid arthritis, so this herbal medicine will be discussed further in chapter 10.

Capsaicin: An Herbal Treatment That Has Been Adopted by Conventional Medicine

Capsaicin is the "hot" in all hot chili peppers, including cayenne peppers. A cream containing capsaicin came on the market less than 10 years ago for the purpose of reducing the pain that follows an attack of shingles. However, it was later found that this cream is also effective for osteoarthritis.

Dorothy's Story

Dorothy's fingers ached so badly from her osteoarthritis that she was having trouble doing simple tasks, like getting the lids off of jars or loading the film into her camera. In frustration, she went to her doctor. His first suggestion was that she try taking high doses of ibuprofen—800 mg 3 times a day.

Dorothy had heard that using anti-inflammatories at high doses over a long time could cause ulcers, and she asked the doctor about this. He agreed that it was true. although he explained that they certainly did not cause ulcers in everyone. He suggested that she just try ibuprofen and see if it bothered her stomach.

She still felt reluctant, so she asked if there was anything else she could try—some kind of herbal remedy, perhaps. Her doctor looked faintly startled at the question. "I don't prescribe

What Is the Scientific Evidence for Capsaicin?

A number of studies have been conducted on people who have used capsaicin creams for various pain syndromes, such as shingles, the pain that follows a mastectomy, and the pain associated with diabetes. Two double-blind studies have been conducted on participants with arthritis (both osteoarthritis and rheumatoid arthritis). It must be noted, however, that it's hard to believe the studies really were double blind, since it's impossible to hide the burning sensation caused by capsaicin!

The largest study involved 70 people who were suffering from osteoarthritis. Half of these participants were treated with a cream containing 0.025% capsaicin; the other half received the same cream without capsaicin.[13] Eighty percent of the participants who used the capsaicin cream reported a reduction in their pain after 2 weeks. The average reduction

herbs," he told her. But because she was obviously so uncomfortable with taking the anti-inflammatories, he thought about it for a while. "There is a cream I could give you to rub on the joints that hurt. It won't provide as much relief as the ibuprofen would, but your arthritis isn't all that severe, so maybe it would help. And it's a proven treatment, not a folk remedy!"

Dorothy thanked him, and took the prescription to have it filled. After she got home, she read the label carefully to see what the active ingredient was. When she saw it, she chuckled to herself. The doctor had given her a pharmaceutical cream called Zostrix. The active ingredient was capsaicin—which Dorothy recognized as the "hot" in hot red peppers! It was an herbal treatment after all.

in pain was 33%. Only two of the people being treated with capsaicin withdrew because of the burning sensation that is the primary side effect of this treatment.

Another double-blind study found similarly positive results.[14]

Despite the small number of controlled clinical trials, the use of capsaicin creams has become an accepted part of medical therapy. This is due in part to the fact that we know how this plant-derived chemical works.

How Does Capsaicin Work?

All sensations from the skin are relayed to the brain. One of the chemicals used by nerve cells that carry the sensation of pain is a small protein called substance P.

Capsaicin causes these nerve cells to release substance P. This release is what produces the characteristic hot, burning sensation you feel when you eat hot peppers. However, when capsaicin is applied continuously for a while, substance P is depleted, and the nerves can't pass along pain signals as efficiently as before. (Actually, this is a somewhat simplified version of a more complicated process.) Other sensory nerves are unaffected, so you will not experience numbing of the area to which the capsaicin is applied. What you will experience is some welcome relief.

You may be asking yourself how applying capsaicin to the skin will help when the pain is coming from the joints beneath the skin. The answer lies in the fact that these nerve cells are branched, with some of the branches supplying the skin and others supplying the structures beneath the skin. Substance P is apparently depleted from all of the branches at the same time, providing relief from the pain of the arthritic joint.

Dosage

Capsaicin-containing creams are widely available in pharmacies. The creams used in the scientific literature contained either 0.025% or 0.075% capsaicin. A recent review article suggests using the higher dosage cream.[15]

When you start out, use only a little cream, as it will produce a burning sensation. After several applications, the burning will begin to diminish. This means that substance P is starting to be depleted. You can then increase the amount of cream you use. When you no longer feel the burning, you then know that you have reached the right dose. (The same method works with hot sauces. If you build up gradually, you will soon be able to painlessly down enough hot peppers to amaze and thrill your friends!)

Safety Issues

Capsaicin creams appear to be safe. The only reported side effect is the initial uncomfortable burning sensation, which stops after a few moments. In the studies, a few people quit using the medication because of this. However, remember that this effect will subside. Of course, you will want to avoid getting capsaicin into your eyes or onto other sensitive tissues. The pain can be quite excruciating, although no real harm should result. Take care to wash your hands after each application, or wear a glove while applying it. If you should need to apply capsaicin to your hands, one manufacturer's recommendation is to apply it for 30 minutes, then wash it off after it has had time to have its effect. Otherwise, you may very well end up rubbing it into your eyes.

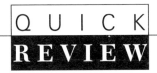

QUICK REVIEW

- All NSAID drugs owe their origin to willow bark.
- Willow bark is a source of salicin, which was turned into aspirin by a German chemist.
- If you use willow bark for pain, keep in mind that it can cause all the same side effects as aspirin, including stomach ulcers, allergic reactions, and Reyes syndrome (a serious kidney disorder that can occur when children take aspirin).
- Willow bark is not recommended for young children or pregnant or nursing women.
- The herb devil's claw is widely used in Europe as a treatment for arthritis of various types. The usual dose is 60 to 800 mg daily of a form standardized to contain to 1 to 3% iridoid glucosides or 1 to 2% harpagoside.

- Boswellia may be useful for osteoarthritis, although it is more often used for rheumatoid arthritis.
- The spicy substance in hot peppers, capsaicin, has become a conventional medical treatment for arthritis. It's available in the form of a cream, and the amount applied should be gradually increased until pain relief is attained.

Essential Fatty Acids (EFAs) for Rheumatoid Arthritis

Perhaps the most common dietary advice you hear these days is to eat less fat. Saturated fats, found in milk, beef, animal products, and certain vegetable oils, certainly do seem to be harmful when taken in excess. Researchers have discovered that these fats increase the incidence of a great many diseases, including the big three killers: cancer, heart disease, and strokes.

However, not all fat is bad. Unsaturated fats seem to be healthy. These include the monounsaturated fats found in olive oil and canola oil as well as the polyunsaturated fats found in other vegetable oils.

Two special types of polyunsaturated fats go even further than this. Not only are they good for you, they seem to be as essential as vitamins. These are called essential fatty acids (EFAs). Just as vitamin C deficiency causes scurvy, severe deficiencies of EFAs can lead to dry skin, hair loss, eczema, decreased immunity, and arthritis.

Evidence gathered over the last two decades suggests that supplemental doses of certain EFAs may be able to

Fish Oil: The Eskimo Connection

The Inuit (Eskimo) people of Greenland eat an enormously high-fat diet, but they don't develop heart disease very often. Curiosity about this led researchers to investigate the fatty acids found in fish and seals, the major foods in their diet. Subsequent research found that these foods contain high levels of omega-3 essential fatty acids, leading to a wave of interest in these substances.

Further investigation showed that the Inuit people also have very little rheumatoid arthritis.[1] This observation led researchers to perform scientific studies on the effectiveness of fish oil for rheumatoid arthritis. As described in this chapter, it really seems to work.

reduce the symptoms of rheumatoid arthritis. However, we have no direct evidence as yet that they can modify the course of the disease, like the DMARD drugs can.

Types of Essential Fatty Acids

Essential fatty acids fall into two major categories: omega-3 and omega-6. There are many fatty acids in each of these groups. Figure 8 shows the relationship between some of the more important members of these two families of fatty acids.

EFAs seem to be as essential to the body as vitamins.

You can think of each of these families as an assembly line. The fatty acids at the top, LA and ALA, are the starting ingredients. Your body then turns on the assembly line and manufac-

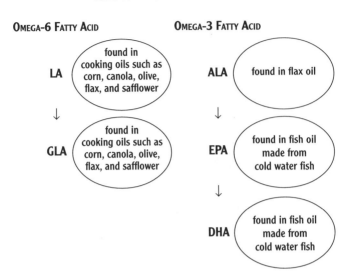

OMEGA-6 FATTY ACID   OMEGA-3 FATTY ACID

LA — found in cooking oils such as corn, canola, olive, flax, and safflower

ALA — found in flax oil

GLA — found in cooking oils such as corn, canola, olive, flax, and safflower

EPA — found in fish oil made from cold water fish

DHA — found in fish oil made from cold water fish

Figure 8. *Omega-3 and omega-6 fatty acids break down into other acids*

tures other fatty acids from them. In the omega-6 family, the body turns LA into gamma linolenic acid (GLA) and then into dihomo-gamma-linoleic acid (DHGLA). In the omega-3 family, the body starts with alpha-linolenic acid (ALA) and makes eicosapentaenoic acid (EPA) and docosahexaenoic acid (DHA) from it.

You can also eat foods that already contain these essential fatty acids. EPA and DHA are found in fish oil made from cold water fish such as salmon, mackerel, and herring. GLA is found in high concentrations in evening primrose oil, borage oil, and black currant oil.

There has been an enormous amount of scientific interest in the medicinal properties of each of these fatty acids. EPA and DHA may reduce the risk of heart attacks. GLA is used to treat symptoms of diabetes, breast soreness that occurs with menstrual periods, and eczema. And all these essential fatty acids may also be useful in rheumatoid arthritis.

Fatty Acids and Rheumatoid Arthritis

The body uses essential fatty acids to make other substances of great importance. If the assembly line shown in figure 8 were continued further, it would show how GLA, EPA, and DHA are all eventually converted into substances called prostaglandins and leukotrienes.

EPA and DHA are found in fish oil made from cold water fish such as salmon, mackerel, and herring.

You may remember from our previous discussions that nonsteroidal anti-inflammatory drugs (NSAIDs) fight inflammation by limiting the production of prostaglandins. It turns out that some prostaglandins and leukotrienes cause inflammation, while others do not cause much inflammation, and still others may actually reduce it.

As you may recall, the pain and swelling of rheumatoid arthritis is largely caused by inflammation. It turns out that eating foods containing essential fatty acids affects your body's production of prostaglandins and leukotrienes. A higher intake of DHA and EPA seems to lead to the production of more favorable prostaglandins and leukotrienes. Because these fatty acids are found in fish oil, this may explain why fish oil appears to be helpful in rheumatoid arthritis. GLA also appears to reduce rheumatoid arthritis symptoms, for reasons that are more complex and less fully understood.

Omega-3 Fatty Acids: Fish Oil

The experience of the Inuit people suggests that a diet high in omega-3 fatty acids can prevent rheumatoid arthritis from starting. We have no direct evidence that the same results will occur in non-Inuit who merely take fish oil capsules. However, good evidence tells us that regular use of fish oil supplements can reduce symptoms of rheumatoid arthritis in people who have already developed the disease. Keep in mind, though, that fish oil may not alter the course of the disease.

What Is the Scientific Evidence for Fish Oil?

The major source of omega-3 fatty acids used in studies of rheumatoid arthritis is fish oil. According to the results of 12 double-blind placebo-controlled studies involving a total of over 500 participants, supplementation with omega-3 fatty acids can significantly reduce the symptoms of rheumatoid arthritis.[2] It seems to do so with minimal side effects.

GLA is found in high concentrations in evening primrose oil, borage oil, and black currant oil.

One double-blind placebo-controlled study of fish oil followed 90 participants with mild to moderately severe rheumatoid arthritis for a full year.[3] The investigators found that supplementation with 2.6 g of omega-3 fatty acids daily led to significant clinical benefit and reduced the need for other drugs.

The participants were randomly assigned to one of three groups. One group received 6 capsules (1 g each) of fish oil per day, for a daily total of 2.6 g of omega-3 oil (1.7 g EPA and 1.1 g DHA). The second group also received 6 capsules, but half contained olive oil, so the total daily dose was lower. The placebo group received 6 capsules containing nothing but olive oil. The results were impressive. By 3 months, participants taking the highest dosage of omega-3s showed significant improvements in pain levels as compared to those taking placebo, and this

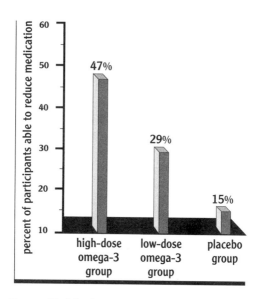

Figure 9. *Double-blind study shows that fish oil may reduce the need for conventional arthritis medications* (Geusens et al., 1997)

improvement continued through the end of the 12-month study. Furthermore, 47% of these participants were able to reduce the dosage of conventional medications that they were taking, compared to only 29% in the low dose omega-3 group and only 15% in the placebo group (see figure 9).

When a study finds that—within an appropriate range—the higher the dose, the greater the improvement, the results are considered especially meaningful. This so-called dose responsiveness tends to mean that a treatment is really working.

The only side effect attributed to fish oil was gastric discomfort. For most participants, this was minor and temporary, and only one person from each group withdrew because of side effects. (Yes, someone in the placebo group developed severe side effects from the treatment!

This always happens. Just as power of suggestion can improve symptoms, it can also cause phantom side effects.)

Other double-blind placebo-controlled studies have also found that participants in the fish oil group could decrease or discontinue their use of conventional medications more successfully than those given a placebo.[4,5,6]

Dosage

For fish oil, the daily dose should supply about 1.7 g of EPA and 0.9 g of DHA. Depending on the product, this may be 6 capsules (1 g each) of fish oil or more a day. Fish oil takes as long as 6 to 12 weeks for the full effect to be noticed.

Some fish oil products contain vitamin E to prevent the essential fatty acids from going rancid. Others are actually sold in oxygen-free capsules to provide the same protection.

Omega-3 oils are abundant in the flesh of cold water marine fish, like salmon, mackerel, and herring. Cod liver oil is another source of omega-3 oils. It is less expensive than the fish oils, but it has the disadvantage of tasting worse. While an

Fish oil takes as long as 6 to 12 weeks for the full effect to be noticed.

emulsified variety of cod liver oil overcomes this problem to some degree, there are still some safety issues as described in the next section of this chapter.

Many people object to the fishy taste and "fish burps" caused by fish oil. Some natural medicine authorities have recommended flaxseed oil as an alternative. Flaxseed oil is rich in the omega-3 fatty acid called alpha linolenic acid (ALA), which, as we've seen, can be converted into EPA in the body. However, in one clinical trial flaxseed oil was found to be ineffective in reducing symptoms or in raising the participants' levels of EPA and DHA.[7] The explanation may be that the conversion from ALA to EPA is very slow and may be impaired in some individuals.

Safety Issues

Fish oil appears to be quite safe. In most of the clinical studies, an upset stomach and other GI symptoms like belching and flatulence were the only side effects. While these reactions may sound rather unappealing, they may be preferable to pain.

However, cod liver oil supplies a great deal of vitamins A and D, two vitamins that can be toxic when taken in excess. **Warning:** Pregnant women particularly must be careful not to take more than 4,000 IU of vitamin A daily because of risks of birth defects.

Because fish oil can "thin" the blood slightly, it may not be safe to combine fish oil with blood thinners such as Coumadin (warfarin), heparin, and perhaps even aspirin. It is even conceivable that fish oil could cause problems if combined with natural products that slightly thin the blood themselves, such as garlic, ginkgo, and high dose vitamin E.

If you are taking any of these medications, seek medical advice before using fish oil. There have also been reports that fish oil can raise cholesterol levels in diabetics, but these have been disputed.[8]

Omega-6 Fatty Acids: GLA

The evidence for GLA is less solid than for the omega-3 fatty acids found in fish oil. However, a few studies suggest that high intake of this essential fatty acid may be helpful for rheumatoid arthritis symptoms.

What Is the Scientific Evidence for GLA?

In a recent double-blind placebo-controlled study, 37 participants received either 1.4 g of GLA (from borage seed oil) or placebo and were followed for 6 months.[9] None of the participants was taking DMARDs. At the end of 6 months, all symptoms of disease activity in the participants taking GLA showed significant improvement. These effects took 6 to 12 weeks to develop. Those taking a placebo stayed the same or got worse. Adverse reactions to GLA in this study included loose stools, flatulence, and belching.

One study showed that the beneficial effects of GLA took 6 to 12 weeks to develop.

A subsequent double-blind placebo-controlled study followed 56 participants given either 2.8 g of GLA daily or placebo for a period of 6 months.[10] In order to deliver this much GLA, a specially concentrated form of borage oil was used. At the end of 6 months, those taking the GLA experienced meaningful and statistically significant improvement in a number of symptoms, including the number of tender joints, the duration of morning tenderness, and the amount of pain. The placebo group did not show any substantial improvement.

Other smaller rheumatoid arthritis studies showed similar benefits.[11,12] Although negative or inconclusive results have also been seen in studies, the overall conclusion appears to be that GLA may offer some benefit for rheumatoid arthritis, especially when combined with standard treatment.[13]

Dosage

According to the studies just described, you may need 1.4 to 2.8 g of GLA daily for optimal benefits. Borage oil, evening primrose oil, and black currant oil all contain some GLA.

Safety Issues

GLA appears to be quite safe. Animal studies suggest that it is nontoxic and noncarcinogenic and does not cause birth defects.[14]

Over 4,000 participants have participated in trials of GLA, primarily in the form of evening primrose oil. No adverse effect has been attributed to this treatment, and in the double-blind placebo-controlled studies of evening primrose oil, there have been no significant differences in rate of side effects between the treated group and the placebo group. In addition, by 1992 over 500,000 prescriptions of evening primrose oil had been issued by the U.K. National Health Service with no significant problems reported.

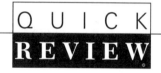

QUICK REVIEW

- Essential fatty acids, like vitamins, must be eaten regularly to provide our bodies with the materials needed for healthy functioning.
- Essential fatty acids fall into two categories: omega-3 and omega-6.
- The omega-3 fatty acids are found in cold water fish, such as salmon, herring, and sardines.
- Omega-6 fatty acids are found in evening primrose oil, borage oil, and black currant oil.

- Essential fatty acids are converted into chemical compounds that influence inflammation. Both omega-3 and omega-6 oils have been found in clinical trials to provide some relief from the pain of rheumatoid arthritis, with the strongest evidence being for fish oil supplements that contain omega-3.

- However, there is no evidence that essential fatty acids can modify the course of rheumatoid arthritis or prevent joint damage.

- Fish oil is slow acting, taking as long as 6 to 12 weeks for the full effect to be noticed. A dose providing at least 1.7 g of EPA and 0.9 g of DHA daily should be used.

- Side effects of fish oil include mild digestive distress and fishy burps, flatulence, and diarrhea.

- The proper dose of GLA appears to be 1.4 to 2.8 g daily; however, it is difficult to get this much from the products available on the market today. Side effects are rare.

Herbs for Rheumatoid Arthritis

A number of herbs may be helpful for rheumatoid arthritis. However, the scientific study of these herbs is still in its infancy. A few were traditionally used to treat conditions that resemble the modern diagnosis of rheumatoid arthritis, while others have anti-inflammatory properties that might make them useful. But we have very little direct evidence that they are effective. The information in this chapter should be considered as a work in progress.

Boswellia

Boswellia serrata is a shrubby tree that grows in the dry hills of the Indian subcontinent. It is the source of a resin called salai guggal, which has been used for thousands of years in Ayurvedic medicine, the traditional medicine of the region. It is very similar to a resin from a related tree, *Boswellia carteri,* otherwise known as frankincense. Both substances have been used for various diseases that involve inflammation, including rheumatoid arthritis and osteoarthritis.[1]

Recent research has identified boswellic acids as the likely active ingredients in either salai guggal or olibanum. In animal studies, boswellic acids have shown interesting anti-inflammatory effects. They appear to reduce inflammation, but unlike NSAIDs, they do not affect prostaglandins (see chapter 4 for a discussion of prostaglandins).[2,3]

What Is the Scientific Evidence for Boswellia?

A recent issue of the reputable scientific journal *Phytomedicine* was devoted entirely to boswellia and briefly reviewed previously unpublished studies on the herb.[4] A pair of placebo-controlled trials involving a total of 81 participants with rheumatoid arthritis found a significant reduction in swelling and pain over the course of 3 months. Furthermore, a comparative study in 60 people over 6 months found the boswellia extract produced symptomatic benefits comparable to oral gold therapy (gold therapy was briefly discussed in chapter 4).

The full effects of boswellia can take 4 to 8 weeks to develop.

However, this review was rather sketchy on details. It did not state whether or not boswellia could induce remission like gold shots, and not enough evidence was given to evaluate the quality of this research.

However, a recent double-blind placebo-controlled study that enrolled 78 patients found no benefits.[5] About half the patients dropped out, which diminishes the significance of the results.

The bottom line: while boswellia appears to be a promising treatment for rheumatoid arthritis, more research is needed.

The Placebo Effect

Many people are willing to accept that a plant has medicinal value solely on the basis of its popular or traditional use, without necessarily demanding the evidence provided by rigorous scientific testing. The reasoning? "If so many people claim it is effective, it must be working; if it has been used for centuries, it must be doing some good." One problem with these arguments is that they don't take into account the power of suggestion.

Over the last several decades, medical researchers have become only too impressed by the power of the placebo effect. "Pills" containing absolutely nothing of medicinal value have been found time and time again to bring about very real improvements in people who believe they are taking medicine. While this is a rather amazing testimonial for the power of our own minds to heal us, it casts considerable doubt on the effectiveness of herbs that have not been compared against placebo in properly performed double-blind studies.

Dosage

The dosage of boswellia most often recommended for rheumatoid arthritis is 400 mg 3 times a day of an extract standardized to contain 37.5% boswellic acids. The full effect is said to take as long as 4 to 8 weeks to develop.

Safety Issues

Few side effects have been reported with boswellia other than an occasional allergic reaction or a mild upset stomach. However, due to the lack of formal safety studies, boswellia is not recommended for young children, pregnant or nursing women, or those with severe liver or kidney disease.

Curcumin

Turmeric, the flavoring and coloring spice derived from the root of *Curcuma longa,* has been used for centuries as a food and a medicine in Indian and Southeast Asian cultures. It is one of the dominant ingredients in red curry sauces.

Turmeric is traditionally believed to have tonic (strengthening) and carminative (gas-relieving) properties. Curcumin, one of the primary constituents of turmeric, has been investigated as a potential anti-inflammatory agent. Curcumin has been found to be a rather potent inhibitor of inflammation in animal tests, affecting the production of both prostaglandins and leukotrienes.[6–10] It is this finding

The study of herbs for rheumatoid arthritis is an area of research still in its infancy.

that is the primary basis for the belief that turmeric may be effective in rheumatoid arthritis. However, it is a long step from animal and test tube studies to results in people. There is not really any direct evidence as yet that turmeric or curcumin are effective for rheumatoid arthritis.

What Is the Scientific Evidence for Curcumin?

There has been one small double-blind study of curcumin for rheumatoid arthritis.[11] This study was designed to compare the effectiveness of curcumin and the older NSAID drug phenylbutazone. Phenylbutazone proved to be more effective.

Nonetheless, symptoms improved in the curcumin group as well. For this reason, this study is often incorrectly cited as evidence that curcumin is an effective treatment for rheumatoid arthritis. It actually doesn't prove anything of the kind. The benefits seen in the curcumin group could simply have been due to the power of suggestion, which can be counted on to produce some effects even with a completely worthless treatment. We really need double-blind studies that compare curcumin to placebo to know whether it is truly effective.

Studies in animals have shown that curcumin can inhibit inflammation.

Still, curcumin is widely used in India as a treatment for rheumatoid arthritis, and physicians there report that it appears to be effective.

Dosage

For the treatment of rheumatoid arthritis, a commonly recommended dosage of curcumin is 400 mg 3 times a day.[12] You would need to take 8 g of ordinary turmeric a day to get that much of curcumin, but products that contain nearly pure curcumin are available.

Safety Issues

Turmeric is a common spice that has been consumed in large dosages over long periods of time by millions of people. It is on the GRAS (Generally Regarded as Safe) list published by the U.S. Food and Drug Administration. However, concentrated curcumin products may present presently unrecognized risks. Safety in young children, pregnant or nursing women, or those with severe liver or kidney disease has definitely not been established.

Bromelain

Bromelain is a protein-digesting enzyme found in the fruit and stem of the pineapple plant, *Ananas comosus.* Pineapple was introduced to Europe following Christopher Columbus's early voyages. It was used as a traditional medicine for a wide variety of ailments throughout South and Central America.

Bromelain was isolated from pineapple juice in 1891. When it was discovered in 1957 that the stem contained more bromelain than the fruit, commercial products containing the isolated enzyme began to be produced.

Bromelain is used in Germany to reduce the swelling caused by surgery and athletic injuries.

What Is the Scientific Evidence for Bromelain?

Studies suggest that bromelain has anti-inflammatory properties,[13,14] and it is commonly used in Germany to reduce the swelling caused by surgery and athletic injuries. These anti-inflammatory properties suggest that bromelain might be effective for rheumatoid arthritis. However, there is as yet no direct evidence that it works.

Dosage

Germany's Commission E recommends that bromelain can be taken at a dosage of 80 to 320 mg daily to reduce the swelling caused by surgery. For rheumatoid arthritis, a dosage of 1,200 to 1,800 mg per day has been recommended.[15] The total dosage is usually divided up for use throughout the day. Bromelain is believed to be best absorbed when taken on an empty stomach.

Safety Issues

Bromelain appears to be quite nontoxic. However, there have been reports of allergic reactions, as well as upset stomach and diarrhea. Bromelain "thins" the blood, reducing its tendency to form clots, and thus should not be combined with other blood-thinning agents such as warfarin (Coumadin), heparin, or perhaps even aspirin.[16] It is also conceivable that bromelain could cause bleeding problems when combined with other natural therapies that mildly thin the blood, such as garlic, ginkgo, and high dose vitamin E. Its safety in young children, pregnant or nursing women, or those with severe liver or kidney disease has not been established.

Ginger

Ginger root is familiar to many people as a spice and flavoring. It is often sliced and served either pickled or candied. It can be consumed as a powdered herb or as a tea. Probably everyone has had ginger ale at some time in their lives, although I'm not sure if there is much ginger in most brands of the modern soda.

In the traditional Ayurvedic medical system of India, as well as the Tibb medical system of ancient Persia, ginger was recommended for rheumatism and inflammation.

Today, it is most widely used to treat nausea and upset stomach (for more information, see _The Natural Pharmacist: Your Complete Guide to Herbs_). However, there is some evidence that ginger may have anti-inflammatory properties.[17,18,19] Again, whether this translates into benefits for rheumatoid arthritis has not yet been determined.

Dosage

When used to treat rheumatoid arthritis, a dosage of 2 to 4 g of powdered ginger daily is commonly prescribed.

This is equivalent to about 20 g of fresh ginger, or about a half-inch slice.

Safety Issues

As a commonly eaten food, ginger is believed to be quite safe, and studies in animals confirm this impression. However, for theoretical reasons, ginger should not be combined with drugs that reduce blood clotting, such as warfarin (Coumadin), heparin, or even aspirin. It is also conceivable that ginger could cause bleeding problems when combined with other natural therapies that mildly thin the blood, such as garlic, ginkgo, and high dose vitamin E. However, no such problems have been reported. The maximum safe dosage of ginger in young children, pregnant or nursing women, or those with severe liver or kidney disease has not been established.

Other Herbs

Devil's Claw

Devil's claw is described in more detail in chapter 8. Evidence suggests that devil's claw can reduce both pain and inflammation, and two double-blind studies found benefits in a variety of arthritic conditions. For details concerning the studies, recommended dosage, and safety of devil's claw, please refer to chapter 8.

Willow Bark

Willow bark has also been discussed in chapter 8. As noted there, willow bark's active ingredient is essentially the same as that of aspirin. For a more detailed overview of the research and safety of willow bark, again, please see chapter 8.

Chinese Thoroughwax

The root of *Bupleurum falcatum* has been used in Chinese and Japanese medicine as a component of formulas whose chief actions are anti-inflammatory and fever reducing. Compounds in the root called saikosaponins have been found to have an anti-inflammatory effect in animals.[20] However, to date, no animal or human studies indicate that this herb is an effective treatment for any kind of arthritis.

Feverfew

Feverfew (*Tanacetum parthenium*) is an herb that has been known since antiquity as a treatment for headaches and arthritis. While there is good preliminary evidence that feverfew may help prevent and reduce the severity of migraine headaches, a study that evaluated its effects in rheumatoid arthritis found no benefit.[21] (For more information, see *The Natural Pharmacist Guide to Feverfew and Migraines*.)

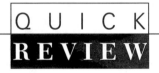

QUICK REVIEW

- Although herbs have long been used to treat many types of arthritis, scientific study of their effectiveness in treating rheumatoid arthritis is fairly new and incomplete.

- Boswellia, a traditional Ayurvedic herb, has some direct evidence to support its use in rheumatoid arthritis. The typical dosage is 1,200 mg per day of a preparation that has been standardized to contain 37.5% boswellic acids.

- Several herbs have anti-inflammatory properties that may make them useful in rheumatoid arthritis. These include curcumin, bromelain, ginger, devil's claw, and Chinese thoroughwax.

- Willow bark may be helpful because it contains aspirin-like substances.
- Evidence suggests that the herb feverfew is not effective for rheumatoid arthritis.

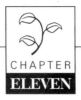

Other Nutrients for Arthritis

I n most cases, vitamins and minerals cannot be made by the human body, but they are essential for the maintenance of good health. A growing body of evidence suggests that vitamin and mineral supplements, or foods that contain them, may be able to help prevent such diseases as cancer and heart disease. Can any of them relieve the symptoms of arthritis, or prevent or slow its progression? The answer is: Well . . . maybe.

This chapter will explain what we know about the effectiveness and safety of these nutritional treatments.

Free Radicals and Antioxidants

Oxygen is essential for life, but it has a dark side. The rust that literally eats holes through an old car is an example of oxygen's ability to cause destruction. In the form of *reactive oxygen species,* oxygen can damage DNA, proteins, glucosaminoglycans, and other large molecules. Molecules containing reactive oxygen or related substances are often called *free radicals,* and the damage they can inflict is called *oxidative damage.* Antioxidants, including vitamins C, E, and beta-carotene (which becomes vitamin A once in your body), help disarm these potentially damaging free radicals.

Free radicals have been implicated in a wide variety of conditions, including cancer, heart disease, cataracts, Alzheimer's disease, and aging itself. It has been suggested that the accumulation of this oxidative damage may contribute to osteoarthritis, rheumatoid arthritis, and other forms of arthritis. If you have felt as though your hinges were rusting, you may not be far from wrong! Antioxidant vitamins, an integral part of the body's defense force against oxidative damage, might play an important role in the prevention and treatment of arthritis of many kinds.

Antioxidant vitamins might play an important role in preventing and treating many kinds of arthritis.

The most important antioxidant vitamins are C, E, and beta carotene. Each of these vitamins serves its own special purposes within the body, but they also work as a team with one another and with the natural defense systems that protect the body. So as we discuss each vitamin or mineral separately, keep in mind that combinations may turn out to be the best way to prevent or treat arthritis.

Vitamin C: May Slow Osteoarthritis

The best evidence for antioxidant vitamins' effects on arthritis can be found for vitamin C. Researchers looked at 640 participants in the Framingham Heart Study over a period of 8 to 10 years to see whether vitamin C or other nutrients made a difference in osteoarthritis.[1] The results

A Note About Research

The most common method for studying the influences of vitamins and minerals is an *observational study*. In such a study, researchers keep track of the vitamin and mineral intake of the participants and monitor certain aspects of their health over a period of many years. Unfortunately, the data from such studies can be misleading.

The problem is that researchers can't know for certain what influences in the participants' lives are most important. For example, people who habitually take in more vitamin C, for example, might also tend to exercise more or eat less fat. A benefit that seems to be due to the vitamin supplement may actually be caused by these other factors. Researchers try to take

---

were impressive. People whose diets provided very little vitamin C showed a rate of worsening of arthritis three times greater than those who received more. This was a highly significant difference. Curiously, high dietary intake of vitamin C did not seem to prevent arthritis from developing in the first place. It just slowed it down.

We really don't know how vitamin C works. In addition to being an antioxidant, vitamin C is necessary for the production of collagen. It is possible, though by no means proven, that in addition to protecting against oxidative damage, vitamin C contributes to maintaining healthy cartilage.

A problem with this study is that it followed total vitamin C taken in the diet, not just vitamin C supplements. Whenever you eat food such as fruits and vegetables that are high in vitamin C, you are also getting lots of other healthful substances, most importantly a group of substances called

everything into account, but it isn't possible to do so perfectly. There is always a certain amount of doubt about the results.

Better studies, called *intervention trials,* actually intervene in patients' lives. In these studies, participants are either given vitamin C or placebo, for example, and then followed for a period of time: the familiar double-blind study. Studies of this type are much more reliable because researchers have more control over what factors are changing in the participants' lives. However, few of these studies have been performed to investigate the effects of vitamins and minerals on arthritis. We have to rely instead on the much less solid results of observational trials. Fortunately, they can still give us some good information.

flavonoids. It's hard to tell whether it was really the flavonoids or actually just the vitamin C that made the difference.

To know whether vitamin C supplements work alone, we really need a double-blind study in which some people are given vitamin C supplements, others are given placebo, and everyone eats approximately the same diet. But no such study has been done.

However, a report of a controlled trial in guinea pigs does provide some corroborating evidence. Like humans, guinea pigs need vitamin C in their diet. The study compared the effect of high dosages (150 mg per day) and low dosages (2.4 mg per day) of vitamin C on the progression of artificially induced arthritis.[2] After 15 to 22 weeks, the arthritis in animals that received the lower dosage of vitamin C showed much more severe changes. Those on high dosages of vitamin showed less cartilage loss.

The Framingham Heart Study

Much of what we know about the role of nutrition in the development and progression of heart disease has come from the Framingham Heart Study, in which 5,200 healthy Americans have been tested every 2 years for signs of heart disease. Started in 1948, and initially intended to last 20 years, the Framingham Heart Study has just celebrated its 50th anniversary. Despite its name, it has been expanded to include information on other diseases, including osteoarthritis.

This is an encouraging sign that supplemental vitamin C might really make a difference in the rate of progression of arthritis. If this preliminary research is backed up by more solid studies in people, vitamin C may turn out to be a chondroprotective drug, as has been hypothesized for glucosamine, chondroitin, and SAMe.

Dosage and Safety Issues

We don't really know the optimal dosage of vitamin C. However, the people in the Framingham osteoarthritis Cohort Study who experienced the greatest protection from the progression of osteoarthritis took in an average of about 500 mg of vitamin C daily from all sources, including food. At this dosage, vitamin C is believed to be entirely safe.

Vitamin E: May Slow Osteoarthritis to a Lesser Extent

The primary function of vitamin E in the body appears to be to protect the cell membrane from free radicals. Of all

Eat Your Fruits and Vegetables

Can vitamin C and a diet high in fruits and vegetables influence arthritis? Let's consider two hikers: Sam and Charles.

Sam and Charles were both diagnosed with knee arthritis at age 60. Charles eats lots of fruits and vegetables and takes a multivitamin supplement every day. Sam rarely eats any vegetables other than French fries and ketchup, avoids fruit, and takes no vitamins. How will they fare in the next few years?

Sam's arthritis may stop him from hiking by age 65. However, according to the results of the Framingham study, Charles might be able to keep on going up till 75—simply because of his diet.

the antioxidants, vitamin E has the best evidence for preventing heart disease and cancer, but it may be useful in arthritis as well. (For more information, see *The Natural Pharmacist Guide to Heart Disease Prevention* and *The Natural Pharmacist Guide to Reducing Cancer Risk.*)

In the Framingham study, high intake of vitamin E was also associated with slower progression of osteoarthritis, although the effect wasn't as dramatic as for vitamin C.

Small studies suggest that vitamin E may also have a direct pain-relieving effect.[3, 4]

Dosage and Safety Issues

We don't know the optimum amount of vitamin E for arthritis, but 400 IU daily is a safe dosage that is commonly recommended for preventing heart disease. However, because even at this moderate dosage vitamin E slightly "thins" the blood, you should not combine it with prescription blood thinners such as warfarin (Coumadin) or heparin.

Beta-Carotene: Apparently Slows Osteoarthritis, but May Not Be Safe

Beta-carotene is the third of the "Big Three" antioxidants. It is also known as pro-vitamin A because the body turns it into vitamin A. Beta-carotene and its chemical cousins, known collectively as the carotenoids, provide a great deal of protection against free radicals. In the Framingham Heart Study, dietary beta-carotene showed more ability to slow the progression of arthritis than vitamin E, but it was less effective than vitamin C.

Again, the Framingham study included beta-carotene from all sources, both food and dietary supplements. Just as with vitamin C, food sources of beta-carotene also include numerous other substances that may be helpful— the whole family of carotenoids—so it is possible some of the benefits seen were due in part to these other nutrients.

Dosage and Safety Issues

Based on the available evidence, it is probably best to take carotenoids in the form of food. Dark, leafy greens and yellow/orange fruits and vegetables, such as spinach, carrots, and cantaloupe, are the best sources. The long-term use of purified beta carotene supplements may be associated with an increased risk of heart disease and certain forms of cancer.[5,6] (See *The Natural Pharmacist: Your Complete Guide to Vitamins and Supplements* for more information.)

Other Vitamins and Minerals That May Help

Other vitamins and minerals may also help osteoarthritis and rheumatoid arthritis. In this section, we'll look at some of the most frequently mentioned.

Boron: May Reduce Symptoms of Osteoarthritis, but Is It Safe?

Boron is a mineral known to be essential for plants, but its necessity for humans has not been established. It is found in fruits and vegetables, and it's estimated that Americans usually eat between 1.7 and 7 mg per day. Weak evidence suggests that boron may help reduce symptoms of arthritis, and it is commonly included in arthritis "formulas" containing other treatments described in this book. However, there are potential safety concerns with boron.

In a small double-blind placebo-controlled trial, 20 participants with different forms of arthritis in a variety of joints were given either boron or placebo.[7] The participants were evaluated after 3 and 8 weeks, according to their report of severity of pain, limitation of movement, and how much acetaminophen they used.

At the end of 8 weeks, 15 participants were still in the trial. Seven of the people taking boron claimed improvement, while only 1 person taking placebo did so. Also, the group taking boron used significantly less acetaminophen over the course of the study than those who were receiving placebo. However, this was a very small study, and the methods used to gauge improvement leave quite a bit to be desired. Further scientific evidence is necessary before boron can be considered a documented treatment for any type of arthritis.

Dosage and Safety Issues

At this point, we would recommend eating plenty of fruits and vegetables to ensure that you receive an adequate level of boron instead of taking it as a supplement. There are concerns that supplemental boron may raise levels of estrogen and perhaps testosterone.[8,9] While at least one study has not found this effect,[10] the consequences of such hormonal changes are potentially worrisome. We would advise caution at the present time. Why not stick to fruits and vegetables? Besides providing boron, as described earlier they also supply other nutrients that can help arthritis. (Not to mention reducing the risk of cancer and heart disease!)

Pantothenic Acid: May Help
Rheumatoid Arthritis but Not Osteoarthritis

Vitamin B5 was named pantothenic acid from the Greek *pantos,* meaning "everywhere," because it is found in so many foods. In 1963, a report appeared in the British medical journal *Lancet* indicating that the level of pantothenic acid in the blood of people suffering from rheumatoid arthritis was significantly lower than that of healthy people.[11] Furthermore, those with lower levels of pantothenic acid experienced more severe symptoms. However, by itself this does not indicate that taking pantothenic acid will reduce symptoms.

High-dose pantothenic acid may help rheumatoid arthritis.

The only real evidence for the use of pantothenic acid as a treatment for rheumatoid arthritis comes from a study published in 1980. Twenty-two doctors in England conducted a double-blind placebo-controlled trial of pantothenic acid supplementation in 94 participants.[12] Most of them had osteoarthritis (63%), but the study included 27 people with rheumatoid arthritis. Those receiving pantothenic acid started with 500 mg per day, but within a week the dose was increased to 2,000 mg per day. The trial lasted 8 weeks.

The results showed no benefit in osteoarthritis participants. Those with rheumatoid arthritis showed significant reductions in duration of morning stiffness, disability, and pain. To my knowledge, further trials have never been conducted. Based on this preliminary information, however, it does appear that further study would be warranted.

Dosage and Safety Issues

The study just described used 2,000 mg of pantothenic acid per day. However, it is possible that lower dosages may be as beneficial, and many physicians who practice nutritional medicine prescribe 1,000 mg per day.[13]

No adverse reactions have been reported due to pantothenic acid. However, the safety of such extremely high dosages in young children, pregnant or nursing women, or those with severe liver or kidney disease has not been established.

Selenium: May Help Mild Rheumatoid Arthritis

Selenium is a mineral that helps the body manufacture a natural antioxidant enzyme called glutathione peroxidase. Recent information suggests that selenium may help reduce the risk of cancer. (For more information, see *The Natural Pharmacist Guide to Reducing Cancer Risk.*)

Individuals with rheumatoid arthritis have lower-than-average selenium levels.[14] For this reason, selenium supplements have been suggested as a treatment for rheumatoid arthritis. However, no benefits were found in a double-blind placebo-controlled study in which 40 participants with severe rheumatoid arthritis were given either placebo or 256 mcg of selenium in enriched yeast daily.[15] The level of selenium did rise dramatically in the subjects' blood and in their red blood cells, but symptoms and signs of arthritis did not improve.

Some benefit was seen in a more recent double-blind study of more mild rheumatoid arthritis, however, so the question remains open.[16]

Dosage and Safety Issues

A typical daily dosage of selenium is 200 mcg. At this dosage, it is believed to be safe. However, maximum safe doses in young children, pregnant or nursing women, or those with severe liver or kidney disease has not been established.

Manganese: No Direct Evidence That It Helps Rheumatoid Arthritis

Manganese is a trace element present in the body and in food. Like selenium, it is used as a "building block" in a number of enzymes, including another antioxidant enzyme called super-oxide dismutase. In Europe, this enzyme, injected into the joints, is used as a treatment for rheumatoid arthritis. Some natural medicine authorities suggest that manganese can raise superoxide dismutase levels and thereby help rheumatoid arthritis indirectly.[17] However there is no direct evidence that taking manganese as a dietary supplement is helpful.

Nonetheless, it has been suggested that 37% of Americans are marginally deficient in manganese,[18] and it certainly makes sense to get enough if only for general health reasons.

Dosage and Safety Issues

A supplemental dosage of 5 mg per day is safe, and should be enough to make sure that you are not deficient in manganese.

Note: People with liver cirrhosis may not be able to eliminate excess manganese.[19] Since a buildup of manganese in your body could lead to health problems, those with this serious condition should not take manganese (or any other supplement) other than on a physician's recommendation.

Zinc: Not Effective for Rheumatoid Arthritis

While levels of zinc have been found to be lower than normal in the blood of patients with both osteoarthritis and rheumatoid arthritis, supplementation does not appear to be beneficial.[20,21,22]

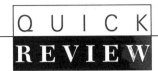

QUICK
REVIEW

- Free radicals (mostly oxygen-containing molecules that can be destructive to parts of our bodies) may play a part in the deterioration of joints in arthritis. Antioxidants, including vitamins A (beta-carotene), C, and E, help protect our tissues from these free radicals.

- Observational and animal studies suggest that dietary vitamin C may slow the rate of deterioration due to osteoarthritis.

- Vitamin E may also slow this deterioration process, though not by as much as vitamin C.

- Beta-carotene from dark, leafy greens and yellow/orange vegetables may be helpful as well.

- The mineral boron may be helpful to those with osteoarthritis, but the evidence now available is too weak to allow us to reach a conclusion, and there are some safety concerns.

- High-dosage pantothenic acid might be helpful for relieving symptoms of rheumatoid arthritis, but further studies are still needed. The usual recommendation is 1,000 mg daily.

- The mineral selenium may be helpful for mild rheumatoid arthritis. The usual dose is 200 mcg daily.

- The minerals zinc and manganese have also been investigated for their potential benefits in arthritis, but so far there is no evidence that they really help.

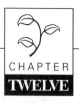

Other Things You Can Do for Arthritis

S o far in this book, you have heard mostly about specific substances such as herbs and supplements. However, your health is influenced by many aspects of your life: Diet, stress levels, exercise, environment, and emotion all play a part in your well-being.

No matter how effective the substances we've discussed might be, they do not operate apart from the rest of your life. It is better to view them as part of a more complete, or holistic, approach to managing your disease process.[1] Elements of this holistic approach certainly include eating a prudent diet, maintaining a proportionate weight for your height, and getting regular exercise. Steps based on ergonomics—the study of using your body efficiently—are also important. For example, you should try to adjust your seat height to keep your knee at approximately a 90-degree angle.

Other nonmedicinal therapies that may be helpful include physical therapy, acupuncture, and the application of magnets. Acupuncture is an ancient Chinese healing art in which very fine needles are placed in specific points to provide pain relief. The use of magnets is an offshoot of acupuncture that comes from Japan.

Education and support is also very important. Learning about your disease and what you can do to improve the situation, as well as addressing the emotional impact that such physical problems can have on you, can make a real difference in how well you will respond to treatment.

Diet for Rheumatoid Arthritis

The idea that changing your diet can positively affect rheumatoid arthritis has been around for a long time. Many different diets have been proposed and popularized, and many books have been written on the subject. Unfortunately, many of these books offer conflicting opinions on what the correct diet for rheumatoid arthritis might be. A small body of scientific research at least lends credence to the idea that changes to the diet can relieve some of the symptoms.

Diet, stress levels, exercise, environment, and emotion all play a part in your well-being.

There is some evidence that vegetarianism, or at least eating large quantities of vegetables, may help rheumatoid arthritis to a certain extent. In one study, 16 participants with rheumatoid arthritis fasted for 7 to 10 days, then followed a lactovegetarian diet (dairy products, but no other animal products such as eggs, fish, or meat) for 9 weeks.[2] Researchers found a statistically significant improvement in a number of measures during the fast. However, symptoms returned when participants began to eat again, even though their diet had been altered. You can't fast forever, so this study was not very encouraging.

A later study of a similar type of diet, however, yielded more positive results. This trial followed 53 participants for 1 year. The 27 participants in the treatment group were admitted to a health resort for 4 weeks, where they fasted for 7 to 10 days, just as in the study above. Then, for the first 3½ months, these participants ate a diet containing no animal-derived foods. They also eliminated foods that contain gluten (such as wheat). For the remainder of the year, they ate a lactovegetarian diet (fruits, vegetables, and dairy products). The control group was admitted to a convalescent home for 4 weeks, but their diet was not altered.

After the first 4 weeks, the diet group showed significant improvement in 10 different symptoms, including significant reduction in pain. The control group's only significant improvement was decreased pain. After 1 year on the special diet, the same symptoms were evaluated again, and the diet group continued to do better than the control group.[3] After this study, additional research was performed to try to understand exactly what it is about this diet that might bring about improvement for rheumatoid arthritis sufferers.

The most obvious explanation is that fruits and vegetables contain high levels of natural antioxidants, including flavonoids, carotenes, and vitamin C. Another theory points out that vegetarians take in more essential fatty acids than nonvegetarians. However, one study designed to examine this possibility found no connection between changes in the amount of fatty acids present in a person's blood and whether they got relief of symptoms by following this diet.[4]

Another suggestion revolves around the finding that changing the diet changes the sort of bacteria that normally lives within our intestines. Researchers checked to see if the intestinal bacteria were altered in any way when people with rheumatoid arthritis used the fasting and diet changes discussed—and they did! This study found that those participants who responded best to the dietary changes also had significantly different bacteria than the participants who did not obtain as much relief on the same diet.[5] These results suggest that, in some cases, the presence of certain types of bacteria may be aggravating rheumatoid arthritis symptoms. If this were the case, then eliminating the food that permits these bacteria to exist would make you feel better. This is not yet proven, but seems to warrant further investigation.

In one study, corn and wheat alone each caused symptoms of rheumatoid arthritis in over 50% of participants.

Another theory holds that immune system responses to chemicals in foods could also cause or exacerbate rheumatoid arthritis. To test this hypothesis, several studies have evaluated various kinds of elimination diets, in which people remove allergenic foods (foods that commonly cause allergies) from their diet. One of the best was a double-blind placebo-controlled study of dietary therapy in 53 participants with rheumatoid arthritis.[6] Over the 6 weeks of the study, those on the diet experienced significant improvement (in pain, stiffness, and number of painful joints, as well as a number of laboratory values used to monitor rheumatoid arthritis) as compared to the control group.

This group of researchers later conducted a study to identify which specific foods could produce symptoms of rheumatoid arthritis.[7] Forty-eight participants went on an elimination diet for 6 weeks, after which certain foods were added back into their diets one at a time. Forty-one of the participants identified foods that caused symptoms. Corn, wheat, pork, oranges, and milk were the most commonly offending foods, and corn and wheat alone each caused symptoms in over 50% of these participants.

If you wish to use this method, you must find the specific foods to which you are reacting. For instance, two reports describe people who got better when a specific food was removed from their diet.[8] In one case the food was milk, and in the other it was corn. In both cases, the participants experienced worsening of their symptoms when the food was reintroduced without their knowledge.

If you wish to try eliminating foods from your diet, seek help. A health-care professional can assess your sensitivity to specific foods and make sure you don't end up with serious nutritional deficiencies.

Weight Reduction for Osteoarthritis

Can losing weight help your arthritis? The results are not conclusive.

One observational study suggested that weight loss can reduce the risk of developing symptomatic osteoarthritis of the knee in women.[9] This seems reasonable, as excess weight increases the stress on the knee joint. However, to date, no studies have tested weight loss as a treatment for osteoarthritis. One study did look at the possibility that the positive results seen in other studies on changes in diet were caused by weight loss, but found no correlation between the amount of weight loss and the improvement of symptoms.

Nonetheless, if you are overweight, you should make every attempt to lose weight. Increased weight is associated with accelerated progression of the disease.[10]

Exercise

It was once thought that exercising a joint with osteoarthritis would cause it to "wear out" faster. Recent evidence, however, suggests that exercise can play a central role in maintaining a healthy joint. Furthermore, research shows that exercises designed to strengthen the muscles surrounding an osteoarthritic joint can lead to improved function and better psychological health.[11] However, the fact that it is difficult, if not impossible, to do "placebo" exercise makes these studies suggestive only.

Exercise can play a central role in keeping your joints healthy.

Two controlled studies on osteoarthritis of the knee have found that strengthening the muscle that straightens the leg (the quadriceps) allows participants to have less disability and possibly less pain.[12] Another couple of studies suggested that a regimen of moderate aerobic exercise, like walking or swimming, also improves the ability to function with osteoarthritis.[13] In one study, which also included stretching and psychological support, physical activity increased by 24% and pain decreased by 14%. The use of medications was also lower. However, because all three elements of the treatment were combined, we don't know if the positive effects were because of the exercise, the stretching, or the psychological support—or all of them.

Both of the studies that included aerobic exercise indicated that participants with moderate to severe osteoarthritis of the knee can benefit from participating in activities equivalent to walking or swimming for 30 minutes 3 times a week.[14] Putting all this information together, it appears that regular exercise should probably be a part of your treatment plan if you develop osteoarthritis.

Consult with your doctor or a physical therapist for recommendations about the type of exercise and its intensity.

Physical Therapy Treatments: Ergonomics, Ultrasound, TENS, Icing, and Heat

Physical therapists offer a number of options that may help arthritis. These can include investigating your work habits to see if it's possible to minimize the stress you put on your body (an ergonomic study), and perhaps relaxing the muscles and tendons surrounding your joints by using ultrasound therapy.

Some physical therapists use transcutaneous nerve stimulation, or TENS, to give temporary relief from pain.

The direct application of heat or cold to an affected joint can provide at least short-term relief. A survey of participants with rheumatoid arthritis and osteoarthritis attending a clinic found that 60% of them used warm baths or other forms of heat applied to the skin. Another 22% liked to apply cold to painful areas.[15] This is certainly a low-cost plan, and it is quite safe as long as you follow the generally recommended procedures: keep a towel between your skin and a cold pack, don't fall asleep on your heating pad, and don't leave either on your skin for a prolonged period of time.

Acupuncture

Acupuncture is a traditional treatment that has been used in Asia for more than 2,000 years. Researchers have conducted a few double-blind placebo-controlled trials on the use of acupuncture to treat osteoarthritis, and two of these were reviewed in an article in the *Annals of Internal Medicine*.[16] Neither study, however, is evidence that acupuncture is effective.

One double-blind trial observed 40 participants with osteoarthritis. The active treatment group received acupuncture at traditional points. The placebo treatment consisted of inserting needles at random points. Treatment was done once a week for 8 weeks. Two physicians who did not know which participants had received which treatments evaluated the results.

Acupuncture is a traditional treatment that has been used in Asia for more than 2,000 years.

Both groups improved to some extent, as would be expected due to the placebo effect. However, the results did not show any difference in outcome between the real acupuncture and the fake acupuncture groups.

Another study compared acupuncture with no treatment. Two groups of 16 participants each received either 20 minutes of acupuncture twice a week for 3 weeks, or no treatment at all. Everyone was evaluated after 9 weeks. Those receiving treatment reported a 23% decrease in pain, compared to a 12% worsening of pain in the untreated group. While this is a very significant result, it is impossible to tell if acupuncture was really beneficial on its own, or if the improvement was a placebo effect from having needles inserted, or simply from receiving attention.

One problem with acupuncture studies is that most of them tend to use a predetermined set of points for the treatment of all participants. True acupuncture, however, is much more sophisticated and individualized to the symptoms of each individual. For this reason, such limited studies cannot fully assess the power of this traditional art.

Magnets

Magnet therapy, an offshoot of traditional acupuncture, is widely used in Japan. Magnets are applied either to the point of pain or to related acupuncture points. It would be very easy to design a double-blind study of magnet therapy, but none have yet been reported.

One double-blind placebo-controlled study looked at the effect of a pulsed electromagnetic field instead of standard magnets. Twenty-seven participants with osteoarthritis received treatment for 30 minutes, 3 to 5 times a week. Participants who received the real magnetic pulses had a 39% reduction in pain, compared with an 8% reduction in those who received the placebo treatment.[17,18]

If properly designed trials of magnets as therapy for arthritis confirm that the treatment was useful, this would be a rather easy and inexpensive device for the control of pain. Additional studies are being planned.[19]

Education and Support

Feeling that you have emotional support can also help you feel better. A recent observational study found that people with rheumatoid arthritis who have supportive marriages and close personal social relationships tended to experience less severe pain than those whose spouses were critical or uninterested or those who had few close friends.[20]

You can also count on yourself for help. Two of the most positive things you can do for yourself are to learn about your disease and take an active role in your own treatment. Several studies, including one randomized trial, have shown that a program of health education to assist with self-management actually reduces pain.[21] In addition, evidence shows that education can reduce health-care costs and produce benefits that last for as long as 4 years.

You can pursue this information in a number of ways: Ask your doctor for information. If you have a computer, you can seek information on the Internet and participate in newsgroups and message boards that focus on your disease. Continue to read books on your illness (like this one!) and magazines that report new findings in health. The more control you take over your own health, it seems, the better you are likely to feel. (**Warning:** Be careful with information found on the Internet, particularly regarding medications. While this book has been carefully reviewed by several health-care professionals to ensure its accuracy, similar screening of information is done on only a few selected Web sites. When in doubt, talk with your doctor before changing any of your medications.)

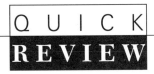

QUICK REVIEW

- In addition to the supplements and drug therapies discussed in this book, there are a number of nonmedicinal approaches to treating arthritis.

- Diet has been found to affect the course of rheumatoid arthritis. Eating a vegetarian diet and eliminating certain foods have proved useful in reducing symptoms.

- Maintaining a weight proportionate to your height may reduce your risk of developing osteoarthritis. No studies have been done on using weight loss to reduce symptoms, but there is evidence that being overweight may accelerate damage from osteoarthritis.

- Strengthening and aerobic exercises may reduce pain and increase joint function.

- Some of the standard physical therapy approaches, such as ultrasound, ergonomics, TENS, and applying heat or cold may be helpful.

- Acupuncture is widely used for arthritis, but as yet there is no evidence that it is effective.

- Magnet therapy is popular in Japan, but again there is as yet no scientific evidence that it is effective.

- Education and emotional support appear to be important parts of an arthritis treatment program, leading to improved pain levels and a sense of well-being.

CHAPTER
THIRTEEN

Putting It All Together

For your easy reference, this chapter contains a brief summary of all the practical information contained in this book. Please refer to earlier chapters for more comprehensive information, including a detailed discussion of safety issues.

There are several well-documented natural treatments for osteoarthritis and a number of promising natural alternatives for rheumatoid arthritis as well. One of the most exciting possibilities for people with osteoarthritis is that the natural treatments may actually alter the course of the disease—slow down the gradual worsening of symptoms that otherwise occurs. A treatment that can do this is called *chondroprotective*. However, we don't yet have definitive evidence that any treatment for osteoarthritis really provides this benefit.

Natural Treatments for Arthritis

Glucosamine sulfate is one of the best-documented alternative treatments for osteoarthritis and is widely used in

Europe. Double-blind studies involving a total of over 1,116 people have found that it can reduce pain and improve mobility. There is reason to believe it may be chondroprotective, but no direct proof as yet exists. The proper dose is 500 mg 3 times daily. Glucosamine is nontoxic and causes very few side effects other than occasional digestive distress. Pain relief usually begins in 2 to 4 weeks and reaches maximum effect in 8 weeks.

Chondroitin sulfate is also widely used in Europe for the treatment of osteoarthritis. Controlled studies involving a total of over 450 participants have found that it can reduce pain and improve mobility. There is also evidence that chondroitin sulfate may slow the progression of the disease. The proper dose of chondroitin sulfate is 400 mg 2 to 3 times daily. Chondroitin appears to be very nontoxic and seldom causes any side effects other than occasional mild stomach upset. Generally, it is sold combined with glucosamine.

According to double-blind studies involving more than 1,000 people, **S-adenosylmethionine (SAMe)** can reduce the symptoms of osteoarthritis as effectively as low doses of anti-inflammatory medications. It may also protect cartilage from damage, although this has not been proven. The usual dose of SAMe is 400 mg 3 times daily. Once symptoms improve (usually at about 4 weeks), the dose can be reduced. A maintenance dose of as low as 200 mg per day may ultimately suffice. SAMe appears to be a very nontoxic substance, but some people develop digestive upset if they take the full dose all at once. To avoid this problem, some experts recommend starting at 400 mg a day, and then working up.

According to 12 double-blind placebo-controlled studies involving a total of over 500 participants, **fish oil** can reduce symptoms of rheumatoid arthritis. However, fish oil is not known to modify the course of rheumatoid arthritis like some standard medications. A typical dose is

6 capsules (1 g each) of fish oil daily. Fish oil takes as long as 6 to 12 weeks for the full effect to be noticed. It may not be safe to combine fish oil with blood thinners such as warfarin (Coumadin) and heparin.

Other Possible Natural Treatments

According to preliminary double-blind studies, the herb **devil's claw** can reduce pain and inflammation in people with various types of arthritis. The recommended dose is 600 to 800 mg of a devil's claw extract (standardized to contain 2 to 3% of iridoid glycosides or 1 to 2% harpagosides) 3 times daily. Devil's claw causes few side effects other than occasional mild digestive distress.

Preliminary evidence suggests that ***Boswellia serrata*** may reduce the pain and swelling of rheumatoid arthritis. A typical dose is 400 mg 3 times a day of an extract standardized to contain 37.5% boswellic acids. The full effect may take as long as 4 to 8 weeks to develop. Few side effects have been reported with boswellia, other than an occasional allergic reaction or a mild upset stomach.

Several other herbs may also be useful for arthritis (either rheumatoid arthritis or osteoarthritis), including **willow bark tea, capsaicin cream, curcumin** (from turmeric), **bromelain** (from pineapple), **ginger root,** and the root of *Bupleurum falcatum* (**Chinese thoroughwax**). The supplements **pantothenic acid** and **selenium** may also be helpful.

A diet high in **vitamin C, vitamin E,** and **beta-carotene** may slow the progression of osteoarthritis. Boron supplements may reduce symptoms of osteoarthritis, but the evidence is weak, and there are significant safety concerns.

Notes

Chapter One

1. Rahad S, et al. Effect of non-steroidal anti-inflammatory drugs on the course of osteoarthritis. *Lancet* 2: 519–522, 1989.

2. Palmoski MJ, et al. Effects of some nonsteroidal antiinflammatory drugs on proteoglycan metabolism and organization in canine articular cartilage. *Arthritis Rheum* 23: 1010–1020, 1980.

Chapter Two

1. Rahad S, et al. Effect of non-steroidal anti-inflammatory drugs on the course of osteoarthritis. *Lancet* 2: 519–522, 1989.

2. Palmoski MJ, et al. Effects of some nonsteroidal anti-inflammatory drugs on proteoglycan metabolism and organization in canine articular cartilage. *Arthritis Rheum* 23: 1010–1020, 1980.

3. Fife RS. Osteoarthritis: epidemiology, pathology, and pathogenesis. In: Klippel, JH, ed. Primer on the rheumatic diseases. Atlanta: Arthritis Foundation, 1997: 216.

4. Rothschild BM. Radiologic assessment of osteoarthritis in dinosaurs. *Ann of Carnegie Museum* 59(4): 295–301, 1990.

5. The Merck manual of medical information. West Point, P.A.: Merck & Co., 1997: 224–225.

6. Weak muscles, painful knees? *N Engl J Med Health News* 3(10): 6, 1997.

7. Lequesne MG, et al. Sports practice and osteoarthritis of the limbs. *Osteoarthritis Cartilage* 5(2): 75–86, 1997.

8. Lane NE. Physical activity at leisure and risk of osteoarthritis. *Ann Rheum Dis* 55(9): 682–684, 1996.

9. Lahr DD. Does running exercise cause osteoarthritis? *Maryland Med J* 45(8): 641–644, 1996.

10. Hamerman D. Clinical implications of osteoarthritis and aging. *Ann Rheum Dis* 54: 82–85, 1995.

11. Felson DT. Do occupation-related physical factors contribute to arthritis? *Baillieres Clinical Rheumatol* 8(1): 63–77, 1994.

12. Quick DC. Joint pain and weather: A critical review of the literature. *Minn Med* 80(3): 25–29, 1997.

Chapter Three

1. Isselbacher KJ, et al. Harrison's principles of internal medicine, 13th edition. New York: McGraw-Hill, 1994: 1648–1655.

2. Ariza-Ariza R, Mestanza-Peralta M, and Cardiael MH. Omega-3 fatty acids in rheumatoid arthritis: An overview. *Semin Arthritis Rheum* 27: 366–370, 1998.

3. Isselbacher KJ, 1994.

4. The Merck manual of medical information. West Point, P.A.: Merck & Co., 1997: 226–230.

5. *N Engl J Med Health News* 3(12): 1–2, 1997.

6. Isselbacher KJ, 1994.

7. Presented at Arthritis Foundation Research Conference, Phoenix, A.Z., June 18–20, 1993.

8. Weyand CM and Goronzy JJ. The molecular basis of rheumatoid arthritis. *J Mol Med* 75(11–12): 772–785, 1997.

9. Isselbacher KJ, 1994.

10. Sany J. Clinical and biological polymorphism of rheumatoid arthritis. *Clin Exp Rheumatol* 12(Suppl. 11): 59–61, 1994.

11. Pope RM. Rheumatoid arthritis: Pathogenesis and early recognition. *Am J Med* 100(Suppl. 2A): 3–9, 1996.

Chapter Four

1. Margolis S and Flynn JA. "Arthritis." *The Johns Hopkins White Papers.* Baltimore, M.D.: Johns Hopkins Medical Institutions, 1998: 42–63.

2. Fries JF et al. Toward an epidemiology of gastropathy associated with nonsteroidal antiinflammatory use. *Gastroenterology* Feb; 96(2 Pt 2 Suppl): 647–655, 1989.

3. Hawkey CJ. The gastroenterologist's caseload: Contribution of the rheumatologist. *Semin Arthritis Rheum* 26(6): 11–15, 1997.

4. Margolis S and Flynn JA, 1998.

5. Rahad S, et al. Effect of non-steroidal anti-inflammatory drugs on the course of osteoarthritis. *Lancet* 2: 519–522, 1989.

6. Towheed TE and Hochberg MC. A systematic review of randomized controlled trials of pharmacological therapy in osteoarthritis of the knee, with an emphasis on trial methodology. *Semin Arthritis Rheum* 26(5): 755–770, 1997.

7. Margolis S and Flynn JA., 1998.

8. "Protecting Against Bone Loss from Steroids." Tufts University Health & Nutrition Letter, Jan. 1998, Vol. 15, No. 11: 7.

9. The Merck manual of medical information. West Point, P.A.: Merck & Co., 1997: 291–292.

10. Weisman MH. Getting tough with rheumatoid arthritis. *N Engl J Med Health News* 3(12): 1–2, 1997.

11. Stucki G, Langenegger T. Management of rheumatoid arthritis. *Curr Opin Rheumatol* 9(3): 229–235, 1997.

12. Hauselmann HJ. Mechanisms of cartilage destruction and novel nonsurgical therapeutic strategies to retard cartilage injury in rheumatoid arthritis. *Curr Opin Rheumatol* 9(3): 241–250, 1997.

13. Margolis S and Flynn JA, 1998.

14. Furst DE. The rational use of methotrexate in rheumatoid arthritis and other rheumatic diseases. *Br J Rheumatol* 36(11): 1196–1204, 1997.

15. Furst DE, 1997.

16. Salaffi F, et al. Methotrexate-induced pneumonitis in patients with rheumatoid arthritis and psoriatic arthritis: Report of five

cases and review of the literature. *Clin Rheumatol* 16(3): 296–304, 1997.

17. Cannon GW. Methotrexate pulmonary toxicity. *Rheumatic Dis Clin North Am* 23(4): 917–937, 1997.

18. Roux N, et al. Pneumocystis carinii pneumonia in rheumatoid arthritis patients treated with methotrexate. A report of two cases. *Rev Rhum Engl Ed* 63(6): 453–456, 1996.

19. Georgescu L, et al. Lymphoma in patients with rheumatoid arthritis: Association with the disease state or methotrexate treatment? *Semin Arthritis Rheum* 26(6): 794–804, 1997.

20. Georgescu L, et al., 1997.

21. Ferraccioli GF, et al. Effects of cyclosporin on joint damage in rheumatoid arthritis. *Clin Exp Rheumatol* 15(Suppl. 17): 83–89, 1997.

22. Fox RI. Mechanism of action of leflunomide in rheumatoid arthritis. *J Rheumatol Suppl* Jul; 53: 20–26, 1998.

23. FDA Press Release. Rockville, Maryland, Sept. 11, 1998.

24. Trentham DE. Dynesius-Trentham rheumatoid arthritis. Antibiotic therapy for rheumatoid arthritis. Scientific and anecdotal appraisals. *Rheum Dis Clin North Am* Aug; 21(3): 817–834, 1995.

Chapter Five

1. Steinman D. "Green Bay Packers choose glucosamine." *Let's Live* (January): 104, 1998.

2. Setnikarr I, et al. Antireactive properties of glucosamine sulfate. *Arzneimittelforschung Drug Res* 41(1): 157–161, 1991.

3. Barclay TS, Tsourounis C, and McCart GM. Glucosamine. *Ann Pharmacother* 32: 574–579, 1998.

4. Noack W, et al. Glucosamine sulfate in osteoarthritis of the knee (abstract). *Osteoarthritis Cartilage* 2: 51–59, 1994.

5. Drovanti A et al. Therapeutic activity of oral glucosamine sulfate in osteoarthrosis: A placebo-controlled double-blind investigation. *Clin Ther* 3(4): 260–272, 1980.

6. Pujalte JM et al. Double-blind clinical evaluation of oral glucosamine sulfate in the basic treatment of osteoarthritis. *Curr Med Res Opin* 7: 110–114, 1980.

7. Vaz AL. Double-blind clinical evaluation of the relative efficacy of ibuprofen and glucosamine sulfate in the management of osteoarthrosis of the knee in out-patients. *Curr Med Res Opin* 8: 145–149, 1982.

8. Muller-Fassbender H, et al. Glucosamine sulfate compared to ibuprofen in osteoarthritis of the knee (abstract). *Osteoarthritis Cartilage* 2(1): 61–69, 1994.

9. Qui, XG, et al. I. Efficacy and safety of glucosamine sulfate versus ibuprofen in patients with knee osteoarthritis. *Arzneimittelforschung Drug Res* 48(1): 469–474, 1998.

10. Crolle G and D'Este E. Glucosamine sulfate for the management of arthrosis: A controlled clinical investigation. *Curr Med Res Opin* 7(2): 104–109, 1980.

11. Drovanti A, et al. Therapeutic activity of oral glucosamine sulfate in osteoarthrosis: A placebo-controlled double-blind investigation. *Clin Ther* 3(4): 260–272, 1980.

12. Pujalte JM, et al. Double-blind clinical evaluation of oral glucosamine sulfate in the basic treatment of osteoarthritis. *Curr Med Res Opin* 7: 110–114, 1980.

13. D'Ambrosio E, et al. Glucosamine sulfate: A controlled clinical investigation in arthrosis. *Pharmatherapeutica* 2: 504–508, 1981.

14. Rovati LC et al. A large, randomized, placebo controlled double-blind study of glucosamine sulfate vs. piroxicam and vs. their associations, on the kinetics of the symptomatic effect in knee osteoarthritis. *Osteoarthritis Cartilage* 2(Suppl. 1): 1994.

15. Forster KK et al. Longer-term treatment of mild to moderate osteoarthritis of the knee with glucosamine sulfate—A randomized, controlled, double-blind clinical study (abstract). *Eur J Clin Pharmacol* 50(6): 542, 1996.

16. Rovati LC. The practical development of a selective drug for osteoarthritis: Glucosamine sulfate. Madrid, Spain: The Ninth Eular Symposium, 1996.

17. Rovati, 1996.

18. Rovati et al., 1994.

19. Forster et al., 1996.

20. Glucosamine for osteoarthritis. *Med Lett Drugs Ther* 39(1010): 91–92, 1997.

21. Setnikarr I, et al. Antireactive properties of glucosamine sulfate. *Arzneimittelforschung Drug Res* 41(1): 157–161, 1991.

22. Basleer C, Henrotin Y, and Franchimont P. In-vitro evaluation of drugs proposed as chondroprotective agents. *Int J Tissue React* 14: 231–241, 1992.

23. Jimenez SA, et al. The effects of glucosamine on human chondrocyte gene expression. Madrid, Spain: The Ninth Eular Symposium, 1996: 8–10.

24. Hellio MP, et al. The effects of glucosamine on human chondrocyte gene expression. Madrid, Spain: The Ninth Eular Symposium, 1996: 11–12.

25. Qui XG, et al., 1998.

26. Lozada CJ and Altman RD. Chondroprotection in osteoarthritis. *Bull Rheum Dis* 46(7): 5–7, 1997.

27. Taphindas MJ, Rivera IC, and Bignamini AA. Oral glucosamine sulfate in the management of arthrosis: Report on a multicenter open investigation in Portugal. *Pharmatherapeutica*, 3(3): 156–168, 1982.

28. Setnikar I. Antireactive properties of "chondroprotective" drugs. *Int J Tissue React* 14(5): 253–261, 1992.

29. Setnikar I, et al. Pharmacokinetics of glucosamine in man. *Arzneimittelforschung* 43: 1109–1113, 1993.

Chapter Six

1. Creamer P and Dieppe PA. Novel drug treatment strategies for osteoarthritis. *J Rheum* 20(9): 1461–1464, 1993.

2. Baici A, et al. Analysis of glycosaminoglycans in human serum after oral administration of chondroitin sulfate. *Rheumatol Int* 12: 81–88, 1992.

3. Conte A, et al. Biochemical and pharmacokinetic aspects of oral treatment with chondroitin sulfate. *Arzneimittelforschung Drug Res* 45: 918–925, 1995.

4. Ronca F, et al. Anti-inflammatory activity of chondroitin sulfate. *Osteoarthritis Cartilage* 6(Suppl. A): 14–21, 1998.

5. Michel, BA. Introduction. *Osteoarthritis Cartilage,* 6(Suppl. A): 2, 1998.

6. Bucsi L and Poór G. Efficacy and tolerability of oral chondroitin sulfate as a symptomatic slow-acting drug for osteoarthritis (SYSADOA) in the treatment of knee osteoarthritis. *Osteoarthritis Cartilage* 6(Suppl. A): 31–36, 1998.

7. Uebelhart D, et al. Effects of oral chondroitin sulfate on the progression of knee osteoarthritis: a pilot study. *Osteoarthritis Cartilage,* 6(Suppl. A): 39–46, 1998.

8. Bourgeois R, et al. Efficacy and tolerability of CS 1200 mg/day vs CS 3x400 mg/day vs placebo. *Osteoarthritis Cartilage* 6(Suppl. A): 25–30, 1998.

9. Morreale P, et al. Comparison of the antiinflammatory efficacy of chondroitin sulfate and diclofenac sodium in patients with knee osteoarthritis. *J Rheumatol* 23: 1385–1391, 1996.

10. L'Hirondel JL. Klinische Doppelblind-Studie mit oral verbreichtem Chondroitionsulfat gegen Placebo bei der tibiofemoralen Gonarthrose. *Litera Rheumatol* 14: 77–84, 1992.

11. Conrozier T and Vignon E. Die Mirkung von Chondroitionsulfat bei der Behandlung der Huftgelenksarthose. Eine Doppelblindstudie gegen Placebo. *Litera Rheumatol* 14: 69–75, 1992.

12. Bucsi L and Poór G, 1998.

13. Verbruggen G, Goemaere S, and Veys EM. Chondroitin sulfate: S/DMOAD (structure/disease modifying anti-osteoarthritis drug) in the treatment of finger joint OA. *Osteoarthritis Cartilage* 6(Suppl. A): 37–38, 1998.

14. Uebelhart D, et al. Protective effect of exogenous chondroitin 4,6-sulfate in the acute degradation of articular cartilage in the rabbit. *Osteoarthritis Cartilage* 6(Suppl. A): 6–13, 1998.

15. Ronca F, et al., 1998.

16. Hungerford DS. Treating osteoarthritis with chondroprotective agents. *Orthop Special Ed* 4(1): 39–42, 1998.

17. Ronca F, et al., 1998.

18. Ronca F, et al., 1998.

19. Hungerford DS, 1998.

20. Bourgeois R, et al., 1998.

21. Ronca F, et al., 1998.

22. Hanson, R. Oral glycosaminoglycans in treatment of degenerative joint disease in horses. *Equine Practice* 18(10): 18–21, 1996.

23. Hungerford DS, 1998.

24. Graedon J and Graedon T. "The People's Pharmacy," *Seattle Times* L4, Aug. 9, 1998.

Chapter Seven

1. Stramentinoli G. Pharmacologic aspects of S-adenosylmethionine. *Am J Med* 83(Suppl. 5A): 35–42, 1987.

2. di Padova C. S-Adenosylmethionine in the treatment of osteoarthritis: Review of the clinical studies. *Am J Med* 83(Suppl. 5A): 60–65, 1987.

3. Caruso I and Peitrogrande V. Italian double-blind multicenter study comparing S-adenosylmethionine, naproxen, and placebo in the treatment of degenerative joint disease. *Am J Med* 83(Suppl. 5A): 66–71, 1987.

4. Bradley JD, et al. A randomized, double-blind, placebo-controlled trial of intravenous loading with S-Adenosylmethionine (SAM) followed by oral SAM therapy in patients with knee osteoarthritis. *J Rheumatol* 21: 905–911, 1994.

5. Maccagno A, et al. Double-blind controlled clinical trial of oral S-adenosylmethionine versus piroxicam in knee osteoarthritis. *Am J Med* 83(Suppl. 5A): 72–77, 1987.

6. Glorioso SS, et al. Double-blind multicentre study of the activity of S-adenosylmethionine in hip and knee osteoarthritis. *Int J Clin Pharmacol Res* 5: 39–49, 1985.

7. Domljan Z, et al. A double-blind trial of ademetionine vs. naproxen in activated gonarthrosis. *Int J Clin Pharmacol Ther Toxicol* 27: 329–333, 1989.

8. Muller-Fassbender H. Double-blind clinical trial of S-adenosylmethionine versus ibuprofen in the treatment of osteoarthritis. *Am J Med* 83(Suppl. 5A): 81–83, 1987.

9. Vetter G. Double-blind comparative clinical trial with S-adenosylmethionine and indomethacin in the treatment of osteoarthritis. *Am J Med* 83(Suppl. 5A): 78–80, 1987.

10. di Padova C, 1987.

11. Berger R and Nowak H. A new medical approach to the treatment of osteoarthritis. *Am J Med* 83(Suppl. 5A): 84–88, 1987.

12. König B. A long-term (two years) clinical trial with S-adenosylmethionine for the treatment of osteoarthritis. *Am J Med* 83(Suppl. 5A): 89–94, 1987.

13. Stramentinoli G, 1987.

14. Harmand MF, et al. Effects of S-Adenosylmethionine on human articular chondrocyte differentiation: an in vitro study. *Am J Med* 83(Suppl. 5A): 48–54, 1987.

15. di Padova C, 1987.

16. di Padova C, 1987.

17. Iruela LM, et al. Toxic interaction of S-adenosylmethionine and clomipramine. *Am J Psych* 150: 522, 1993.

18. Laudanno OM, et al. Complete cytoprotective action on the gastroduodenal mucosa induced by SAMe against damage provoked by ethanol in man. *Panminerva* Med 29: 75–78, 1987.

19. di Padova C, 1987.

20. di Padova C, 1987.

Chapter Eight

1. Solecki RS and Shanidar IV. A neanderthal flower burial in Northern Iraq. *Science* 190: 880–881, 1975.

2. Abelson PH. Medicine from plants. *Science* 247: 513, 1990.

3. Akerele O. The best of both worlds: Bringing traditional medicine up to date. *Soc Sci Med* 24(2): 177–181, 1987.

4. Weissman G. Aspirin. *Sci Am* (January): 84–90, 1991.

5. Schulz V, et al. Rational phytotherapy. New York: Springer-Verlag, 1998: 144.

6. Newall C. Herbal medicines: a guide to health-care professionals. London: Pharmaceutical Press, 1996: 268–269.

7. ESCOP Monographs, Fascicule 2, *Harpagophyti radix,* 1996: 1.

8. ESCOP, 1996: 4.

9. ESCOP, 1996: 4.

10. Mussard C, et al. A drug used in traditional medicine, *Harpagophytum procumbens:* no evidence for NSAID-like effect on whole blood eicosanoid production in human. *Prostaglandins Leukotrienes Essential Fatty Acids* 46: 283–6, 1992.

11. ESCOP, 1996: 5.

12. ESCOP, 1996: 4.

13. Deal CL et al. Treatment of arthritis with topical capsaicin: A double blind trial. *Clin Ther* 13: 383–395, 1991.

14. McCarthy GM and McCarty DJ. Effect of topical capsaicin in the therapy of painful osteoarthritis of the hands. *J Rheumatol* 19: 604–607, 1992.

15. Fusco BM and Giacovazzo M. Peppers and pain: The promise of capsaicin. *Drugs* 53(6): 909–914, 1997.

Chapter Nine

1. Ariza-Ariza R, Mestanza-Peralta M, and Cardiael MH. Omega-3 fatty acids in rheumatoid arthritis: an overview. *Semin Arthritis Rheum* 27: 366–370, 1998.

2. James MJ and Cleland LG. Dietary n-3 fatty acids and therapy for rheumatoid arthritis. *Semin Arthritis Rheum,* 27: 85–97, 1997.

3. Geusens P, et al. Long-term effect of omega-3 fatty acid supplementation in active rheumatoid arthritis. *Arthritis Rheum* 37(6): 824–829, 1994.

4. Skoldstam L, et al. Effect of six months of fish oil supplementation in stable rheumatoid arthritis: a double-blind, controlled study. *Scand J Rheumatol* 21: 178–185, 1992.

5. Lau CS, Morley KD, and Belch JJ. Effects of fish oil supplementation on non-steroidal anti-inflammatory drug requirement in patients with mild rheumatoid arthritis: a double-blind placebo controlled study. *Br J Rheumatol* 32: 982–989, 1993.

6. Kremer JM. Effects of modulation of inflammatory and immune parameters in patients with rheumatic and inflammatory disease receiving dietary supplementation of n-3 and n-6 fatty acids. *Lipids* 31(Suppl): 243–247, 1996.

7. Nordström DCE, et al. Alpha-linolenic acid in the treatment of rheumatoid arthritis: A double-blind placebo-controlled and randomized study. *Rheum Int* 14: 231–234, 1995.

8. Harris WS. Dietary fish oil and blood lipids. *Curr Opin Lipidol* 7: 3–7, 1996.

9. Leventhal LJ, Boyce EG, and Zurier RB. Treatment of rheumatoid arthritis with gamma-linoleic acid. *Ann Intern Med* 119: 867–873, 1993.

10. Zurier RB, et al. Gamma-linolenic acid treatment of rheumatoid arthritis. *Arthritis Rheum* 39(11): 1808–1817, 1996.

11. Leventhal LJ, Boyce EG, and Zurier RB. Treatment of rheumatoid arthritis with blackcurrant seed oil. *Brit J Rheumatol* 33: 847–852, 1994.

12. Leventhal LJ, Boyce EG, and Zurier RB, 1993.

13. Rothman D, et al. Botanical lipids: Effects on inflammation, immune responses and rheumatoid arthritis. *Sem Arthritis Rheum* 25: 87–96, 1995.

14. Horrobin DF. Nutritional and medical importance of gamma-linolenic acid. *Prog Lipid Res* 31: 163–194, 1992.

Chapter Ten

1. Ammon HPT. Salai Guggal — Boswellia serrata: From a herbal medicine to a specific inhibitor of leukotriene biosynthesis. *Phytomedicine* 3(1): 67–70, 1996.

2. Singh GB and Atal CK. Pharmacology of an extract of Salai Guggal ex-*Boswellia serrata,* a new non-steroidal anti-inflammatory agent. *Agents Action* 18: 407–412, 1986.

3. Wildfeuer A, et al. Effects of boswellic acids extracted from a herbal medicine on the biosynthesis of leukotrienes and the course of experimental autoimmune encephalomyelitis. *Arzneimittelforschung* 48(6): 668–674, 1998.

4. Etzel R. Special extract of Boswellia serrata in the treatment of rheumatoid arthritis. *Phytomedicine* 3(1): 67–70, 1996.

5. Sander O, Herborn G, and Rau R. Is H15 (resin extract of Boswellia serrata, "incense") a useful supplement to established drug therapy of chronic polyarthritis? Results of a double-blind pilot study. (English Abstract Only) *Z Rheumatol* 57(1): 11–16, 1998.

6. Flynn DL and Rafferty ML. Inhibition of 5-hydroxy-eicosatetraenoic acid (5HETE) formation in intact human neutro-

phils by naturally-occurring diarylheptanoids: inhibitory activities of curcuminoids and yakuchinones. *Prostaglandins Leukotr Med* 22: 357–360, 1986.

7. Ammon HPT and Wahl MA. Pharmacology of Curcuma longa. *Planta Medica* 57: 1–7, 1991.

8. Aurora R, et al. Anti-inflammatory studies on Curcuma longa (turmeric). *Indian J Med Res* 59: 1289–1295, 1971.

9. Ghatak N, et al. Sodium curcuminate as an effective anti-inflammatory agent. *Indian J Exp Biol* 10: 235–236, 1972.

10. Satoskar RR, et al. Evaluation of anti-inflammatory property of curcumin (diferuloyl methane). *Indian J Med Res* 71: 632–634, 1980.

11. Deodhar SD, et al. Preliminary studies on antirheumatic activity of curcumin. *Indian J Med Res* 71: 632–634, 1980.

12. Lininger S, ed. The natural pharmacy. Rocklin, C.A.: Prima Publishing, 1998: 315.

13. Taussig SJ and Batkin S. Bromelain, the enzyme complex of pineapple (Ananas Comosus) and its clinical application: An update. *J Ethnopharmacol* 22: 191–203, 1988.

14. Schulz, V et al. Rational phytotherapy. New York: Springer-Verlag, 1998: 263.

15. Murray M. Healing power of herbs. Rocklin, C.A.: Prima Publishing, 1996: 68.

16. Schulz V, et al. 1998.

17. Kiuchi F, et al. Inhibitors of prostaglandin biosynthesis from ginger. *Chem Pharm Bull* 30: 754–757, 1982.

18. Kiuchi F, et al. Inhibition of prostaglandin and leukotriene biosynthesis by gingerols and diarylheptanoids. *Chem Pharm Bull* 40: 387–391, 1992.

19. Srivastasva KC. Isolation and effects of some ginger components on platelet aggregation and eicosanoid biosynthesis. *Prostaglandins Leukot Med* 25: 187–198, 1986.

20. Yamamoto M, Kumagi A, and Yamamura Y. Structure and actions of saikosaponins isolated from *Bupluerum falcatum* L. *Arzneim.-Forsch* 25(7): 1021–1023, 1975.

21. Pattrick M, Heptinstall S, and Doherty M. Feverfew in rheumatoid arthritis: a double blind, placebo controlled study. *Ann Rheum Dis* 48(7): 547–549, 1989.

Chapter Eleven

1. McAlindon TE, et al. Do antioxidant micronutrients protect against the development and progression of knee OA? *Arthritis Rheum* 39: 648–656, 1996.

2. Schwartz ER. The modulation of osteoarthritic development by vitamins C and E. *Int J Vit Nutr Res* 26: 141–146, 1984.

3. Machtey I and Ouaknine L. Tocopherol in osteoarthritis: A controlled pilot study. *J Am Geriatr Soc* 26: 328–330, 1978.

4. Edmonds SE, et al. Putative analgesic activity of repeated oral dosages of vitamin E in the treatment of rheumatoid arthritis. Results of a prospective placebo-controlled double-blind trial. *Ann Rheum Dis* 56(11): 649–655, 1997.

5. Albanes D, et al. Effects of a-tocopherol and b-carotene supplements on cancer incidence in the Alpha-Tocopherol Beta-Carotene Cancer Prevention Study. *Am J Clin Nutr* 62(Suppl.): 1427–1430, 1995.

6. Omenn GS, et al. Effects of a combination of beta-carotene and vitamin A on lung cancer and cardiovascular disease. *N Engl J Med* 334: 1150–1155, 1996.

7. Newnham RE. Essentiality of boron for healthy bones and joints. *Environ Health Perspect* 102(Suppl. 7): 83–85, 1994.

8. Nielsen FH, et al. Effect of dietary boron on mineral, estrogen, and testosterone in postmenopausal women. *FASEB J* 1: 394–397, 1987.

9. Naghii MR and Samman S. The effect of boron supplementation on its urinary excretion and selected cardiovascular risk factors in healthy male subjects. *Biol Trace Elem Res* 56(3): 273–286, 1997.

10. Beattie JH and Peace HS. The influence of a low-boron diet and boron supplementation on bone, major mineral and sex steroid metabolism in postmenopausal women. *Br J Nutr* 69: 871–884, 1993.

11. Barton-Wright EC and Elliott WA. *Lancet* 2: 862, 1963.

12. General Practitioner Research Group. Calcium pantothenate in arthritis conditions. *Practitioner* 224: 208–211, 1980.

13. Lininger S, ed. The natural pharmacy. Rocklin, C.A.: Prima Publishing, 1998: 116.

14. Tarp U, et al. Low selenium level in severe rheumatoid arthritis. *Scan J Rheumatol* 14: 97–101, 1985.

15. Tarp U, et al. Selenium treatment in rheumatoid arthritis. *Scand J Rheumatol* 14: 364–368, 1985.

16. Peretz A., et al. Adjuvant treatment of recent onset rheumatoid arthritis by selenium supplementation: preliminary observations. *Br J Rheumatol* 31: 281–286, 1992.

17. Murray M. Encyclopedia of nutritional supplements. Rocklin, C.A.: Prima Publishing, 1996.

18. Freeland-Graves JH, Bales CW, and Behmardi F. Manganese requirements of humans. In: Kies C, ed. Nutritional bioavailability of manganese. Washington, D. C.: American Chemical Society, 1987: 90.

19. Lininger S, ed. The Natural pharmacy. Rocklin, C.A.: Prima Publishing, 1998: 184.

20. Milanino R, et al. Copper and zinc status in rheumatoid arthritis: studies of plasma erythrocytes, and urine, and their relationship to disease activity markers and pharmacological treatment. *Clin Exp Rheumatol* 11(3): 271–281, 1993.

21. Dore-Duffy P, et al. Zinc profiles in rheumatoid arthritis. *Clin Exp Rheumatol* 8(6): 541–546, 1990.

22. Mattingly PC and Mowat AG. Zinc sulphate in rheumatoid arthritis. *Ann Rheum Dis* 41: 456–457, 1982.

Chapter Twelve

1. Griffin MR, et al. Practical management of osteoarthritis: Integration of pharmacologic and nonpharmacologic measures. *Arch Fam Med* 4: 1049–1055, 1995.

2. Skoldstam L, et al. Effects of fasting and lactovegetarian diet on rheumatoid arthritis. *Scand J Rheumato* 8(4): 249–255, 1979.

3. Kjeldsen-Kragh J, et al. Controlled trial of fasting and one-year vegetarian diet in rheumatoid arthritis. *Lancet* 338(8772) : 899–902, 1991.

4. Haugen MA, et al. Changes in plasma phospholipid fatty acids and their relationship to disease activity in rheumatoid arthritis patients treated with a vegetarian diet. *Br J Nutr* 72(4): 555–566, 1994.

5. Peltonen R, et al. Changes of faecal flora in rheumatoid arthritis during fasting and one-year vegetarian diet. *Br J Rheumatol* 33(7): 638–643, 1994.

6. Darlington LG. Placebo-controlled, blind study of dietary manipulation therapy in rheumatoid arthritis. *Lancet,* I: 236–238, 1986.

7. Darlington LG, et al. Dietary manipulation therapy in RA. In: Machtey I, ed. Progress in rheumatology III. Petah-Tiqva, Israel: Rheumatology Service, Golda Medical Center, 1987: 125–132.

8. Darlington LG and Ramsey NW. Review of dietary therapy for rheumatoid arthritis. *Br J Rheumatol* 32: 507–514, 1993.

9. Felson DT, et al. Weight loss reduces the risk for symptomatic knee osteoarthritis in women. The Framingham study. *Ann Intern Med* 116: 535–539, 1992.

10. Hochberg MC. Osteoarthritis: Clinical features and treatment. In: Klippel JH, ed. Primer on the rheumatic diseases. Atlanta: Arthritis Foundation, 1997.

11. Puett DW and Griffin MR. Published trials of nonmedical and noninvasive therapies for hip and knee osteoarthritis. *Ann Intern Med* 121(2): 133–140, 1994.

12. Puett DW and Griffin MR, 1994.

13. Puett DW and Griffin MR, 1994.

14. Puett DW and Griffin MR, 1994.

15. Darlington LG and Ramsey NW. Review of dietary therapy for rheumatoid arthritis. *Br J Rheumatol* 32: 507–514, 1993.

16. Puett DW and Griffin MR, 1994.

17. Puett DW and Griffin MR, 1994.

18. Valbona C, Hazlewood CF, and Jurida G. Response of pain to static magnetic fields in postpolio patients: a double-blind pilot study. *Arch Phys Med Rehabil* 78(11): 1200–1203, 1997.

19. Altman LK. "Study on using magnets to treat pain surprises skeptics." *New York Times,* Dec. 9, 1997.

20. Waltz M, Kriegel W, and van't Pad Bosch P. The social environment and health in rheumatoid arthritis: marital quality

predicts individual variability in pain severity. *Arthritis Care Res* 11(5): 356–374, 1998.

21. Griffin MR, et al. Practical management of osteoarthritis: Integration of pharmacologic and nonpharmacologic measures. *Arch Fam Med* 4: 1049–1055, 1995.

Index

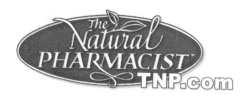

About the Authors

Ron Hobbs, N.D., is dean of the University of Bridgeport College of Naturopathic Medicine. Dr. Hobbs graduated from Bastyr University and is a consulting faculty member for the Institute for Creative Development in Seattle, Washington. He has lectured extensively on the history and philosophy of natural medicine, botanical medicine, and environmental issues.

Gloria Bucco is president of Gloria Bucco & Associates, a creative copywriting firm specializing in newsletters, brochures, and marketing materials that focus on natural health. She is also an independent journalist.

About the Series Editors

Steven Bratman, M.D., medical director of Prima Health, has many years of experience in the alternative medicine field. A graduate of the University of California at Davis, Medical School, he has also trained in herbology, nutrition, Chinese medicine, and other alternative therapies, and has worked closely with a wide variety of alternative practitioners. He is the author of *The Natural Pharmacist: Your Complete Guide to Herbs* (Prima), *The Natural Pharmacist: Your Complete Guide to Illnesses and Their Natural Remedies* (Prima), *The Natural Pharmacist Guide to St. John's Wort and Depression* (Prima), *The Alternative Medicine Ratings Guide* (Prima), and *The Alternative Medicine Sourcebook* (Lowell House).

David J. Kroll, Ph.D., is a professor of pharmacology and toxicology at the University of Colorado School of Pharmacy and a consultant for pharmacists, physicians, and alternative practitioners on the indications and cautions for herbal medicine use. A graduate of both the University of Florida and the Philadelphia College of Pharmacy and Science, Dr. Kroll has lectured widely and has published articles in a number of medical journals, abstracts, and newsletters.